REPRODUCTIVE RIGHTS AND TECHNOLOGY

LIBRARY IN A BOOK

REPRODUCTIVE RIGHTS AND TECHNOLOGY

Rachel Kranz

Facts On File, Inc.

Reproductive Rights and Technology

Facts On File, Inc.
132 West 31st Street
New York NY 10001

Library of Congress Cataloging-in-Publication Data
Kranz, Rachel.
     Reproductive rights and technology / Rachel Kranz.
       p. cm. — (Library in a book)
    Includes bibliographical references and index.
    ISBN 0-8160-4546-1
     1. Human reproductive technology. 2. Human reproductive technology—
Law and legislation. I. Title. II. Series.
    RG133.5 .K73 2002
    616.6'9206—dc21   2001042897

Facts On File books are available at special discounts when purchased in bulk quantities for businesses, associations, institutions, or sales promotions. Please call our Special Sales Department in New York at (212) 967-8800 or (800) 322-8755.

You can find Facts On File on the World Wide Web at http://www.factsonfile.com

Text design by Ron Monteleone

Printed in the United States of America

MP Hermitage 10 9 8 7 6 5 4 3 2 1

This book is printed on acid-free paper.

This book is dedicated to Sally and Tess.

I salute your courage.

Let's hope it won't be necessary again.

CONTENTS

PART III
APPENDIX

ACKNOWLEDGMENTS

With thanks to Robert Jaffe and Cristina Page for their kind assistance.

PART I

OVERVIEW OF THE TOPIC

CHAPTER 1

AN OVERVIEW OF REPRODUCTIVE RIGHTS AND TECHNOLOGY

THE SCIENCE OF REPRODUCTIVE RIGHTS AND TECHNOLOGY

BASIC ANATOMY

For any aspect of reproductive rights and technology to make sense, the basics of reproduction must be understood. This section will review that information, which may be supplemented by a health textbook or basic book on reproduction.

The Female Reproductive System

A woman's contribution to reproduction begins with her eggs (ova), which are contained within her ovaries, two small organs on either side of the lower pelvis. A woman's ovaries are formed while she is still a fetus, during her mother's first trimester of pregnancy. The ovaries of a six-month-old fetus already contain millions of potential eggs, known as germ cells. Some of these germ cells will eventually develop into eggs; others will dissolve and be absorbed back into the body. A baby girl has 2 to 4 million germ cells in her ovaries; a girl at puberty has fewer than half a million. A woman who never becomes pregnant and has regular periods until she reaches menopause will have produced 300 to 400 eggs over her lifetime. The rest of the germ cells will be reabsorbed into her body.

Within each ovary, immature eggs—known as oocytes—are stored within follicles. On day 1 of the menstrual cycle—the first day of menstruation—approximately 20 follicles begin to prepare for ovulation, triggered by the body's release of GnRH (gonadotropin-releasing hormone). GnRH in turn sets off the release of FSH (follicle-stimulating hormone), which stimulates one—or sometimes more—follicles to get ready for ovulation. (If multiple follicles each produce an egg, the woman may become pregnant with multiple fetuses, although multiple births may also result from the separation of the fertilized egg later in the process.)

Over the next two weeks, FSH causes the chosen follicle(s) to produce the hormone known as estrogen, which in turn causes the uterine lining to thicken. On day 14 of the menstrual cycle, the follicle suddenly produces a new quantity of estrogen. This hormonal signal sets off a surge of luteinizing hormone (LH), which finally triggers the follicle to release its egg. That release begins the process known as ovulation.

During ovulation, one or more eggs move into the fallopian tube, a long, thin vessel that connects the ovaries to the uterus (womb). It is during this journey that an egg might be fertilized. If around this time semen (liquid containing sperm) is released in or near the vagina during unprotected intercourse, sperm will attempt to swim up through the cervix (the narrow opening between vagina and uterus) and into the woman's uterus and fallopian tubes. If a sperm encounters an egg within the fallopian tubes, the egg may be fertilized.

The next two weeks are known as the luteal phase. During this time, the now-empty follicle starts to release progesterone, a hormone that causes the endometrium (uterine lining) to thicken. This thick lining will be necessary to nourish a fertilized egg, should pregnancy occur. If there is no fertilized egg, this lining will eventually be shed in the monthly bleeding known as menstruation. Menstruation is set off by hormones known as prostaglandins, which also stimulate the contractions of the uterus that are felt as menstrual cramps.

What if an egg has indeed been fertilized during its journey through the fallopian tube? In that case, the egg and sperm together form a zygote, or embryo, whose cells begin to multiply. Two to three days after fertilization, the embryo has 16 cells and is known as a morula (from the Latin word for "mulberry," since it looks like a cluster of berries). Four or five days after fertilization, the embryo leaves the fallopian tube and enters the uterus. By this point, it is a blastula, two layers of cells surrounding a cavity filled with fluid.

Five or six days after ovulation, the embryo attaches itself to the thickened, premenstrual endometrium. This process is known as implantation, during which enzymes secreted by the embryo break down the cells on the endometrium's surface so that the embryo can burrow underneath. The endometrium then closes over the embryo, covering it completely.

The part of the embryo that is buried most deeply will become the placenta. The other part of the embryo will become the fetus. (During pregnancy, the placenta nourishes the fetus.) After approximately 40 weeks (in the ideally healthy pregnancy), the fetus passes from the uterus through the cervix and out the vagina to be born as a child.

Female Infertility

Clearly, a number of things can go wrong along this journey, making it difficult or impossible for a woman to become pregnant—the condition known as female infertility. A woman may have hormonal problems that keep the cycle from occurring properly. There may be problems in the ovaries or fallopian tubes, so that eggs are not properly released, do not move properly through her system, or are not accessible to sperm. The mucus found at the opening of the cervix may react badly to the sperm seeking to enter. Or the woman may have uterine problems that make it difficult for an embryo to implant itself in her uterine lining.

Some women who are technically fertile—capable of getting pregnant—may have uterine, hormonal, or chromosomal difficulties that prevent a fetus from growing properly, coming to term, or being born.

Reproductive technology has been developed to address a range of female concerns, including preventing pregnancy, terminating pregnancy, and overcoming infertility or uterine difficulties to achieve pregnancy and birth.

The Male Reproductive System

Whereas the female's body contains ova from before birth, the male's body does not begin producing sperm cells until puberty (sexual maturity, usually occurring around age 13). And while a woman is born with all the eggs she will ever have, a man continues to create sperm to replace the ones lost through ejaculation. Sperm are also far more numerous than eggs: An adult female has fewer than half a million eggs, whereas a fertile male releases millions of sperm each time he ejaculates.

Sperm is created with the help of some of the same hormones that are involved in female ovaluation: GnRH, FSH, and LH. The testes also produce testosterone, the male hormone involved in sperm development.

Sperm cells are produced in the testicles or testes, two small (two-inch-diameter) organs located within the scrotum, a loose pouch of skin hanging behind the penis. Sperm must be produced at about 95 degrees Fahrenheit, a temperature slightly below body temperature. Hence, the scrotum is located outside the man's body.

Each testicle is partly covered by the epididymis, where sperm continually mature and where mature sperm are stored. A tube known as the vas deferens (also known as the ductus deferens) connects the epididymis to the prostate gland. During ejaculation, sperm pass from the epidiymis through the vas deferens and into the prostate.

Just below the prostate lie the bulbourethral glands (also called Cowper's glands). Both the prostate and the bulbourethral glands produce fluid as the sperm passes through.

From the prostate gland, semen moves into the man's urethra, which is also connected to the bladder and is used to transport urine out of the body. During ejaculation, however, a nerve reflex closes the bladder's opening, so that urine can not flow out.

The urethra is contained within the penis, spongy tissue that is full of tightly packed blood vessels. When a man becomes sexually aroused, the smooth muscle of the penis relaxes, compressing the blood vessels, so that the penis fills with blood. It is this blood that causes the penis to be stiff, hard, and erect.

When the man reaches orgasm, or ejaculates, his penis releases semen, which contains sperm and various fluids. Sixty percent of semen is seminal fluid, secreted by the seminal vesicles, small glands that lie just behind the bladder.

In unassisted reproduction, a man contributes to fertilization by ejaculating semen into a woman's vagina (or in the close vicinity of her vagina). The semen contains sperm that "swim" up the woman's vagina, through her cervix, into her uterus, and then into her fallopian tubes. If sperm is present when an egg is traveling through the fallopian tube, the sperm may fertilize an egg, beginning the process of pregnancy.

Male Infertility

Clearly, this system, too, may malfunction in a variety of ways. A man may have trouble producing sperm (even if he is producing large quantities of semen); produce sperm that is not able to move properly through the female system; have difficulty achieving or maintaining an erection; have problems in the testes or vas deferens; or have problems with ejaculation. As with an infertile woman, an infertile man may have no trouble performing sexually, and his infertility may go unnoticed until he wishes to have a child.

Reproductive technologies have also been developed to deal with male reproductive concerns, including preventing pregnancy and overcoming infertility. However, even though males share biological responsibility for pregnancy and fertility equally with women (40% of all infertility is attributed to men; 40% to women; 10% is shared; and 10% unexplained), the reproductive technologies available to men are vastly fewer, less advanced, and less invasive than those available to women.

CONTRACEPTIVE TECHNOLOGIES

Contraceptive technologies have existed for thousands of years. Folk wisdom, midwives, and the physicians of ancient civilizations all made their contributions to contraceptive technology. Over the centuries, women and men have used such devices as linen or snakeskin condoms, dried fish powder, sea sponges, and even a mixture of cow dung mixed with honey, which women placed inside their vaginas. (Of course, no one should try these methods today; besides being far less effective than modern contraception, they could have potentially deadly side effects.)

Today's scientists can even give modern scientific explanations for some of these old methods. For example, one ancient form of birth control was to soak some cotton in lemon juice and place it in the vagina; the acid in the lemon would make the vagina more hostile to sperm, serving as a kind of natural spermicide. Queen Anne's lace, or wild carrot, a popular herbal form of birth control, was studied in the 1980s and found to block the production of progesterone and inhibit fetal and ovarian growth in mice. (Again, women today should avoid these methods, as scientists know far too little about either their effectiveness or their safety.)

Another long-used method of birth control was colloquially called "the rhythm method" and known more formally as "periodic abstinence" or FAMs (Fertility Awareness Methods). This method consists of having intercourse only on the days when a woman is not ovulating, because only on those days can she become pregnant. Over the years, various technologies have been used to calculate "safe" days for a woman to have sex, including counting days from the first day of the menstrual cycle and watching for changes in cervical mucus.

Today, the technology most recommended is a thermometer, as a woman's body temperature rises when she ovulates. However, these changes in body temperature vary from woman to woman and may be as small as half a degree Fahrenheit. Moreover, for measurements to be reliable, the temperature must be taken at the same time each day, ideally, first thing in the morning, before the woman has gotten out of bed.

In addition, studies have shown that various factors can suddenly stimulate ovulation in some women, especially teenagers. Sexual activity itself, particularly orgasm, has been known to trigger ovulation. In that sense, there are no "safe" days to have unprotected sex; that is, there is no truly reliable way to predict when pregnancy is possible and when it is not.

Over the years, modern industry, cutting-edge science, and some old folk wisdom have co-existed—often uneasily—to create a number of different reproductive technologies.

Condoms

Condoms have been used for centuries, although the modern form of latex or plastic condom, considered the most reliable, has only been around for a few decades.

The technology behind the condom is simple: The sheath fits around the man's penis and collects the semen when he ejaculates, preventing it from reaching the woman's vagina and impregnating her. Condoms have also been made in a small, caplike form, to fit only over the tip of the man's penis, but these were more likely to slip off than the sheathlike condom (and were considered less comfortable by most men).

Today, condoms are considered most reliable when used in conjunction with a spermicide, such as nonoxynol-9, which may be able to immobilize any sperm that escapes if the condom leaks, breaks, or comes off. Although spermicide is placed inside some condoms, women wishing to prevent pregnancy are generally advised to use a spermicidal foam, cream, jelly, film, or suppository when their male partner uses a condom, whether or not the man's condom also contains spermicide.

(Until recently, condoms plus spermicide were also considered the only effective protection against sexually transmitted diseases during vaginal [penis to vagina] and anal [penis to anus] intercourse. However, United Nations research scientists studying the effectiveness of nonoxynol-9 and other spermicides in Africa have discovered that no known spermicide is effective in preventing HIV [the virus that causes AIDS], and in some cases, uses of large quantities of nonoxynol-9 may even increase women's chances of contracting HIV. The U.S. Centers for Disease Control now recommends the use of condoms, either with or without nonoxynol-9, for HIV prevention.)

In the early 1990s, a female condom was developed: a sheath to be inserted inside the vagina, with a ring at the top that fits around the cervix. Medical studies have found female condoms less effective at preventing disease and pregnancy than male condoms, partly because a man's penis may be inserted inside the vagina but outside the condom and because the cervical ring does not always stay in place. (Users of both sexes have also complained about comfort.)

Spermicides

A spermicide is a substance that immobilizes sperm, preventing it from reaching the woman's fallopian tubes. A woman may insert spermicide into her vagina in the form of foam, jelly, cream, film, or suppository (a small object containing medication, meant to be inserted into the vagina or anus and dissolve there, releasing the medication). In ancient times, vaginal suppositories contained acacia gum, which probably acted both as a spermicide and as a way of sealing up the cervix so that sperm could not pass through. Today's spermicides—in whatever form—eventually dissolve in the vagina.

Diaphragms

Diaphragms, which are made of rubber and fitted over the woman's cervix, are the descendants of many older forms of birth control that sought to physically (rather than chemically) prevent sperm from reaching the cervix. Former versions of the diaphragm have been made of metal, wood, and glass.

The modern diaphragm is a small rubber device shaped like a round, shallow bowl. The concave part of the diaphragm, usually filled with spermicide, fits over the cervical opening. The diaphragm prevents pregnancy in two ways: the rubber device blocks the cervix (the opening to the uterus) and prevents sperm from entering there, and the spermicide immobilizes sperm.

A doctor fits a woman with the proper diaphragm size for her body. Women should be refitted if they gain or lose 10 or more pounds; if they have had a baby, abortion, or miscarriage after 14 weeks of pregnancy; and if they have had abdominal or pelvic surgery.

Once the diaphragm is in position, suction usually helps to keep it in place, although it might be displaced by vigorous intercourse (especially when the woman is on top) or when the woman has a bowel movement. Diaphragms may also tear or crack, allowing sperm to pass through. In theory, spermicide compensates for any movement or tearing in the diaphragm, but pregnancies may occur.

A diaphragm may be inserted up to six hours before intercourse, must be left in place for several hours (to insure that any sperm left in the woman's system continues to be prevented from reaching her cervix), and may be left in place for up to a total of 24 hours. A couple having sex more than once leaves the diaphragm in place and uses a plastic plunger to insert another dose of spermicide into the woman's vagina each additional time they have intercourse.

Some women report discomfort with the diaphragm; others experience irritation and/or infection from the spermicide or in reaction to the rubber. For many, however, it is a highly convenient and effective forth of birth control, and it may actually reduce the risk of cervical cancer.

Cervical Cap

Another barrier method is the cervical cap. This device is smaller and deeper than the diaphragm but also fits over the cervix. It, too, blocks sperm from entering the cervix and contains spermicide to immobilize sperm.

The cervical cap may be left in place for up to 48 hours and does not require the insertion of additional spermicide for repeated sexual encounters. Some women have reported irritation and discomfort with the cervical cap.

It has also raised some concerns about cervical cancer. For many women, however, it is a comfortable and effective form of birth control.

Cervical Sponge

This device is not available in the United States but it can be purchased elsewhere. It was taken off the U.S. market when many women reported developing allergic reactions, irritations, and infections. Although some reports of increased toxic shock syndrome (a severe medical condition in women, associated with the use of tampons) had been associated with the sponge, these reports were later discredited. The sponge is now being readied for return to the U.S. market, although FDA approval has been slower than expected. The sponge, too, has a long history: In ancient times, women used sea sponges, which they placed over their cervix, perhaps soaked in lemon juice or vinegar as a spermicide. Today's sponges also contain spermicide. They prevent conception both by entrapping the sperm and through their spermicidal effect.

Intrauterine Device (IUD)

The IUD is a small, flexible plastic device—usually a T-shaped form about 3 centimeters long—that contains copper or a hormone that it releases. Available by prescription only, an IUD is inserted by a doctor into the uterus and can be left there for up to 10 years, if it contains copper; for up to one year, if it contains the hormone progestin, a form of progesterone, which helps prevent pregnancy by suppressing ovulation and thickening the cervical mucus, preventing sperm from entering the uterus. A doctor must also remove the IUD, which restores fertility immediately. The IUD is the world's most widely used form of women's reversible birth control.

The IUD works in rather mysterious ways. It seems to prevent eggs from being fertilized, but scientists are not sure exactly why. Apparently, it affects the movement of the sperm or egg; or perhaps it releases chemicals that create a hostile environment to sperm. Another theory is that the IUD stimulates the egg to move through the fallopian tube too quickly to be fertilized.

IUDs that contain copper prevent pregnancy in two more ways: The copper affects the enzymes in the uterine wall to prevent implantation, and it stimulates an increased production of prostaglandins, which causes the uterus to contract and reject implantation.

IUDs that contain progestin have three contraceptive effects: They thicken the cervical mucus, suppress ovulation, and stimulate the uterine wall to reject implantation.

IUDs have various side effects and contraindications, though many women use them with ease. Side effects may include heavy menstrual flow, cramps, expulsion of the IUD, uterine puncture, infection, and infertility. It is also possible for an IUD to shift position and become ineffective in preventing pregnancy (although a string attached to the IUD offers women a chance to check their IUDs for position).

Some antiabortion activists and philosophers consider the IUD an abortifacient (something that causes an abortion) rather than contraception (something that prevents conception), because by preventing implantation, the IUD may lead to the destruction of a fertilized egg—although in almost all cases, the IUD has first prevented an egg from being fertilized. However, in some religious and philosophical views, life begins at the moment that the sperm fertilizes the egg, as opposed to the standard medical view, in which life begins at implantation. Thus, by some religious definitions, an IUD might sometimes be considered an abortifacient. Standard medical definitions, however, consider the IUD a contraceptive device.

Birth Control Pills ("The Pill")

There are two types of birth control pill: combinations of estrogen and progestin and progestin-only pills. The combination type suppresses ovulation and may also work to thicken cervical mucus, creating a barrier that sperm cannot cross. Progestin-only pills can also prevent ovulation, but they usually work by thickening the cervical mucus, preventing the sperm from entering the uterus. Both types of pill can prevent fertilized eggs from implanting in the uterus (and so would again be considered abortifacients in some religious definitions).

The side effects of the early pills were quite severe. Today's pills contain 20% less estrogen and more than 10% less progestin than the earlier versions, leading to a dramatic decrease in side effects. However, common side effects still include many symptoms: nausea (and, rarely, vomiting), cramps, bloating, light bleeding during the menstrual cycle, a lighter menstrual flow than usual, breast changes (enlargement, tenderness, secretions), changes in weight, changes in sexual desire, migraine, and depression. Birth control pills also may interact badly with various prescription medications. Women who smoke, have high blood pressure, have had breast or uterine growths, have high cholesterol levels, have liver problems, or have some diabetes-related conditions should not take the Pill. Women taking other medications may need to avoid the Pill. Serious side effects may include blood clots in the legs, lungs, heart, or brain.

Generally, women need to work closely with their doctors to find the hormonal dosage that is right for them. The Pill may offer some protection against infection of the fallopian tubes (PID, or pelvic inflammatory disease, a leading cause of infertility); ectopic (tubal) pregnancy (in which a fertilized egg begins to grow into a fetus within the fallopian tube rather than the uterus); noncancerous breast growths; ovarian cysts or cancer; cancer of the uterine lining; menstrual cramps; acne; and premenstrual symptoms, including headache and depression.

Depo-medroxyprogesterone Acetate (DMPA, Depo-Provera, "the Shot")

Depo-Provera is a prescription-only artificial hormone that resembles progesterone, taken by injection. One shot of Depo-Provera can prevent pregnancy for 12 weeks by suppressing ovulation and thickening the cervical mucus. During the first five days of menstruation, protection is immediate; otherwise, protection begins in two weeks.

Side effects may include irregular bleeding, lighter periods (most women have no periods at all after five years of use, and it may take a year for periods to return after use is stopped), longer or heavier periods, and a range of less common side effects, including increased appetite, weight gain, headache, sore breasts, nausea, nervouness, dizziness, depression, rashes, hair loss, increased facial or body hair, and changes in sex drive. Depression is one potential serious side effect of "the Shot," along with severe vaginal bleeding, breast lumps, severe and sudden abdominal pain, and yellowing of the skin or eye.

Although "the Shot" is considered reversible, it may take 12 months for women to regain fertility, and side effects may continue for up to eight months.

Levonorgestrel Implants (Norplant)

Another progestin-based contraceptive is Norplant, a set of six thin, flexible plastic sticks—about the size of matchsticks—that are surgically inserted under the skin, usually in the upper arm. While they remain in the woman's body, they are effective for five years. They must be surgically removed; after removal their effects will disappear in a few days.

The sticks contain a form of progestin known as levonorgestrel, which resembles the progesterone made by a woman's ovaries. The sticks release a steady stream of the hormone, which suppresses ovulation and thickens the cervical mucus. Norplant may also keep fertilized eggs from implanting in the uterine wall.

Some women should not use Norplant or should use it only under medical supervision. More than 80% of all Norplant users report changes in their menstrual cycles, such as irregular periods, longer and heavier periods, spotting between periods, or no periods at all for months at a time. Other less common side effects include headache, change in appetite, weight gain or loss, depression, dizziness, nervousness, sore breasts, nausea, changed sex drive, decreased vaginal lubrication, acne and skin irritations, gain or loss of facial hair, and in rare cases, enlarged ovaries or ovarian cysts.

An Overview of Reproductive Rights and Technology

Emergency Forms of Contraception

Emergency contraception is, as its name suggests, recommended only in case of an emergency: if a woman has had unprotected sex with a man (including having been raped), or if her method of contraception has failed. Emergency contraception prevents either fertilization or implantation, so the medical community considers it contraception—the prevention of conception—rather than an abortifacient (a means of inducing an abortion, or the termination of an already conceived fetus). (The so-called abortion pill, RU-486 [mifepristone], is discussed below, under Abortion Technologies.) Some people in the pro-life movement may consider emergency contraception to be a form of abortion because it may in some cases prevent a fertilized egg from implanting.

Emergency contraceptive pills, also known as "morning-after" pills, are available in two forms, both resembling ordinary hormonal birth control pills: a combination of estrogen and progestin, and progestin-only.

Despite the colloquial name, an emergency contraceptive pill can be taken any time up to 72 hours after unprotected sex, with a second dose taken 12 hours after the first one. A woman must take the same kind of pill both times. Pills may have side effects, including nausea, for which many doctors recommend antinausea medication. After taking the pills, a woman may experience changes in her next period, nausea, vomiting, breast tenderness, irregular bleeding, fluid retention, and headaches. Emergency contraception may not prevent an ectopic pregnancy.

Another form of emergency contraception involves the insertion of an IUD. Within five days of unprotected sex, a doctor may insert a copper IUD, which can either be left in place for up to 10 years or removed after the next menstrual period (or any time in between).

Sterilization

Female sterilization is known as tubal ligation. It involves sealing off the fallopian tubes so that sperm cannot reach the egg and pregnancy cannot occur. Male sterilization is known as vasectomy. In this procedure, a tiny portion of the vas deferens on each side of the scrotum is removed and the two ends of the vas are sealed with sutures, clips, or electrical current. For more on reversal of these procedures, see Fertility Technologies.

ABORTION TECHNOLOGIES

Abortion is defined as the termination of pregnancy before birth, with the resulting death of the embryo or fetus. A spontaneous abortion, also called a miscarriage, occurs when the pregnant woman has an accident or disorder that prevents her from carrying to term or when the fetus has a disorder that prevents it from developing normally and results in its demise. An induced abortion, by contrast, is caused intentionally, either for health reasons or because the pregnancy is unwanted. An induced abortion may also be called a therapeutic abortion.

Induced abortions may themselves be of two types: elective (by choice), which is the term used when a woman's life or physical health are not immediately at risk; and emergency. Many laws distinguish between elective and emergency abortion, but there is no medical difference between the two procedures. Likewise, there are laws that speak of the "endangerment" of the fetus that do not distinguish between induced and spontaneous abortions.

Like contraception, abortion has a centuries-old history and has been used by folk healers, midwives, and physicians in all parts of the world for thousands of years. Women have also induced their own abortions. Until recently, abortions were high risk for the woman and were often uncertain undertakings that might not effectively end the pregnancy. (For more on the history of abortion, see The History of Reproductive Rights and Technology.)

There are several methods by which an induced abortion can be performed. The most important consideration in choosing the type of abortion has to do with how long the pregnancy has gone on, and thus, how old the fetus is. Gestational age—the age of the fetus—is calculated based on the first day of the woman's last menstrual period. A healthy singleton pregnancy lasts 39 to 40 weeks; multiple pregnancies tend to last for a shorter time.

The 39 to 40 weeks of pregnancy are divided into three periods known as trimesters. The first trimester lasts for 13 weeks; the second runs from week 14 to week 24; the third trimester begins in week 25 and continues until birth. Generally, a viable fetus—one that can survive outside the womb— needs to be at least 25 weeks old, although recent advances in medical science have enabled doctors to save babies born at somewhat earlier ages.

Some 90% of all U.S. abortions are performed during the first trimester, before 12 weeks gestational age. Abortions performed during the first trimester actually pose fewer risks to a woman's health than giving birth: only 0.4 women out of 100,000 die from abortions performed at 8 weeks or earlier, as compared to 1 in 13,000 women who die from giving birth. The mortality rate (rate of people who die) for a first-trimester vacuum aspiration abortion, for example, is about 5 to 10 times lower than the mortality rate of carrying a fetus to term.

Some 10% of all abortions are performed during the second trimester, from week 12 to week 24. Abortions during the early part of the second trimester also pose fewer health risks for the mother than completing a pregnancy. After the second trimester begins, the risks to the mother from an abortion is believed to increase by about 30% per week. Thus, when an abortion takes place at 20 weeks, the mortality rate is 10.4 women per 100,000; at 21 weeks, the rate is 1 in 6,000.

Mifepristone (RU-486) and Misoprostol

A woman who is seven weeks pregnant or less can abort a fetus by taking a combination of two drugs in pill form. The woman begins by taking mifepristone (RU-486), which was approved by the FDA in 2000, although it had been available in Europe several years earlier. Mifepristone blocks progesterone, a hormone needed to mantain the pregnancy. About 48 hours after taking mifepristone, the woman takes misoprostol, a prostaglandin that causes the uterus to contract and expel the fetus.

Misoprostol can also be used in conjuction with methotrexate, a drug originally used to fight cancer because of its interference with cell division. A pregnant woman is injected with methotraxate by a physician, who then prescribes misoprostol to induce uterine contractions and expel the fetus.

Both of these procedures effectively terminate pregnancies about 95% of the time. Women should expect cramping and bleeding, though pain medication can be provided. A side effect may be nausea. In some rare cases, women may experience potentially fatal heart and lung problems.

Preemptive Abortion and Early Uterine Evacuation

Preemptive abortion and early uterine evacuation are similar procedures, the first of which can be performed in the first 4 to 6 weeks of pregnancy, the second of which can be conducted in the first 6 to 8 weeks. In both procedures, a cannula, or narrow tube, is attached to a suction device, like a syringe, and inserted through the cervix into the uterus. The suction device extracts the contents of the uterus, including the embryo. Preemptive abortion uses a smaller cannula. Neither procedure requires anesthesia and both can be performed on an outpatient basis. The most common side effect of preemptive abortions is infection. Early uterine evacuation may lead the woman to bleed heavily for a few days.

Vacuum Aspiration

When a woman is 6 to 14 weeks pregnant, vacuum aspiration is used. It begins by dilating (enlarging) the cervix. Dilators—tapered instruments—may be used to open the cervix, progressing from one slightly larger dilator to the next. A cannula attached to an electrically powered pump is inserted into the uterus, and the pump is used to remove the contents of the uterus. The uterine lining may also be scraped with a curette (a spoonlike tool) to loosen tissue and eventually remove it. This procedure is called curettage. This procedure requires only local anesthesia and may be performed in a clinic or doctor's office. The cervix may sustain minor bruises or slight injuries.

Dilation and Curettage (D&C)

This procedure may be used during the sixth to sixteenth weeks of pregnancy. As the name suggests, the cervix is dilated and then the uterine lining is scraped with a curette. This procedure requires general anesthesia and must be performed in a clinic or hospital. Complications may include reactions to the anesthetic and cervical injuries. Once the most commonly used abortion procedure, D&C has been far less used since the development of vacuum aspiration.

Dilation and Evacuation (D&E)

Abortions become far more difficult after the first 16 weeks of pregnancy, because of the increased size of the fetus and the thinner uterine walls, which stretch as the fetus grows. D&E requires that the cervix be dilated further than in the other procedures just described. Then suction and a large curette are used to remove matter from the uterus, along with a large forceps used to grasp and extract the fetus. D&E must be performed under general anesthesia in a clinic or hospital. It is the most commonly used form of second-trimester abortion; along with a modified form of vacuum aspiration used in the second trimester, it accounts for about 95% of all abortions performed between weeks 12 and 20. It is typically performed during the first weeks of the second trimester, but considered safe up to week 24.

Between weeks 13 and 15, D&E is similar to vacuum aspiration, except that the cervix must be dilated more widely to allow surgical instruments to remove larger pieces of tissue. After week 15, the fetus may need to be dismembered before it can be removed. After 20 weeks, the fetus may be injected with intrafetal potassium chloride or digoxin to cause fetal demise before the fetus is evacuated.

Induction Abortion

This method may be used between week 16 and week 24. A small amount of amniotic fluid, the fluid surrounding the fetus, is extracted from the womb and replaced with another fluid. From 24 to 48 hours later, the uterus begins to contract in response to the new fluid, and the fetus is expelled. When the procedure was first developed, saline (salt) solution was used; today another possibility is a solution that contains prostaglandins (which induces uterine contractions) or pitocin, a synethetic version of the human hormone oxytocin, used to induce labor. Complications may include heavy bleeding, infection, and cervical injuries. This procedure must be performed in a hospital with a stay of one or more days.

Hysterotomy

Abortions performed at the end of the second trimester and the beginning of the third trimester are considered major surgery and are usually only performed when there is a severe fetal problem that might compromise the fetus's chance to survive after birth or when the woman's life or health are gravely at risk. In hysterotomy, the uterus (hysterium) is cut open and the fetus is removed surgically, in a procedure similar to a caesarean section (though with a smaller incision). A hysterotomy is considered major abdominal surgery and is performed under general anesthesia.

Dilation and Extraction (D&X)

In this procedure, the woman's cervix is dilated, the fetus is drawn out partway through the vaginal canal, feet first, and suction is used to remove the brain and spinal fluid from the fetal skull. The skull is then collapsed so that the fetus can be completely removed from the uterus. In this case, too, the fetus may be dismembered as it is pulled through the cervix, so that it can be removed. This procedure has been inaccurately termed "partial-birth abortion" and was the topic of the Supreme Court decision *Stenberg v. Carhart* (See chapter 2).

FERTILITY TECHNOLOGIES

About 40% of all couples' infertility problems have to do with the man involved; 40% with the woman; 10% are shared; and 10% are not able to be diagnosed. However, the vast majority of fertility technologies—and the most invasive and technologically advanced approaches—involve women. This section begins with a brief discussion of male infertility and the medications developed to deal with it and proceeds to a more extensive look at the range of reproductive technologies.

Male Infertility

Male infertility generally comes from infection, hormone imbalance, injury, or anatomical abnormalities. The most common reason for male infertility is a problem with sperm production: either low numbers of sperm (oligospermia, fewer than 4 million sperm in the semen from one ejaculation) or no sperm at all (azoospermia). This might be caused by testicular disease, including infections from such common diseases as mumps, which, when contracted after puberty, can lower or obliterate a man's sperm count. It may also be caused by environmental toxins, which some suspect are the reason that U.S. men are generally producing about one-third less sperm per cubic centimeter of ejaculate than they were in 1929. (See Chronology, chapter 3) A man can retain all other normal sexual functions, which are the result of the hormone testosterone, even if he is not producing normal amounts of sperm.

A man with no sperm count may need to rely upon a sperm donor. A man with low sperm count may be able to fertilize a partner's egg with some kind of assisted insemination or with some form of in vitro fertilization. (See below for more information on all of these options.)

Other sperm-related problems include inadequate motility (ability to move) of sperm or too many abnormal sperm.

In some cases, low sperm counts or other sperm problems are the result of hormonal disorders, and they can be addressed by medications. However, for most men with sperm problems, hormonal therapy is not a solution.

Another rare cause of male infertility is abnormality in the male reproductive tract, such as a varicocele (varicose veins above one or both testicles, which may reduce fertility); an obstruction of the duct system within the male reproductive tract, blocking the outflow of sperm; hypospadias (the abnormal positioning of the opening of the penis on the underside of the penis instead of at the tip); or cryptorchidism (an undescended testicle). Surgery may be able to correct these conditions, but fertility may be impaired even after surgery.

If male infertility results from an infection of the male reproductive tract, treating the infection may restore fertility. Likewise, when radiation and/or chemotherapy are used to treat cancers of the male reproductive tract, fertility may resume some time after treatment has stopped. Few medical solutions are available for men whose fertility is not restored after an infection or a chemical radiation treatment.

Ejaculation disorders are another source of male infertility. Again, very little reproductive technology exists to respond to these disorders. However, impotence (difficulty in achieving or maintaining an erection) may be treated with sildenafil (Viagra), which, after its March 1998 FDA approval, quickly became one of the top-selling drugs on the U.S. market.

Viagra works by increasing the blood flow to the penis in response to sexual stimulaton. During a chemically unassisted erection, the smooth (involuntary) muscles in the penis relax. (These muscles are known as involuntary because they're not under the conscious control of the mind.) This relaxation—an expansion of the muscle—actually compresses small blood vessels, trapping the blood and causing the penis to stiffen. Viagra increases the levels of some of the chemicals involved in the relaxation of that smooth muscle, so that blood flows more freely into the penis tissue that becomes erect. Viagra does not cause erections without sexual stimulation, but when a man is stimulated, the drug is likely to make his erections occur more frequently, last longer, and be firmer. The drug is taken orally from half an hour to four hours before intercourse, with a limit of once a day. It poses serious risks to some patients, particularly those who have heart conditions or who are taking certain other medications.

Ovulation Induction and Hormone Treatments

If a woman's infertility is caused by a problem with ovulation, doctors usually begin at the simplest and least invasive end of the technology spectrum. First, doctors will help a woman determine when she is ovulating, so the couple can time intercourse to the days when she is most fertile. The simplest technology to determine ovulation is the thermometer, as some women's body temperature rises markedly on the mornings of the days of ovulation. Women may also buy kits sold over the counter to measure levels of luteinizing hormone, the hormone whose blood levels peak sharply during ovulation; or a clinic can measure hormone levels. In some cases, ultrasound may be used to detect the presence of mature follicles.

If a woman isn't ovulating properly, she can take medication that stimulates her ovaries to produce more ova and follicles. This is known as ovulation induction. Perhaps the greatest risk of ovulation induction is multiple pregnancy, for if a woman is producing more eggs than usual, the chances increase that more than one egg will be fertilized, resulting in twins, triplets, or higher-order pregnancies (four or more fetuses). A responsible doctor will monitor a woman's egg production when she is taking ovulation medication and warn the couple to use birth control or to avoid intercourse during the months when more than one or two eggs become available.

The best-known drug given to women to help induce ovulation is clomiphene citrate (Clomid). Clomid both stimulates the ovaries to produce multiple follicles (and thus, more eggs) and induces the ovaries to release the eggs—to ovulate.

There is an alternate method of inducing ovulation: injecting a woman with hormones known as gonadotropins, which can be either naturally derived or synthetic forms of follicle-stimulating hormone (FSH). FSH is produced naturally by the pituitary gland; its role is to trigger a follicle to mature. When a woman is injected with extra doses of FSH, her ovaries generally produce multiple follicles. The doctor uses ultrasound to track when one or more mature follicles have formed in the ovaries. Then the woman is injected with a different hormone, human chorionic gonadotropin (hCG), which triggers ovulation—the release of an egg—a day or two later.

This hormonal approach has a higher success rate than Clomid, but it takes more time and involves more discomfort and expense, given the need for daily injections and frequent ultrasounds and blood tests. The hormones also cost more than Clomid. And if the treatment does not work the first time, the entire expensive and uncomfortable process must be repeated— sometimes several times.

A possible side effect of gonadotropins is ovarian hyperstimulation syndrome (OHSS), which causes the ovaries to become enlarged and tender. In some cases, women are hospitalized with this condition, but it can usually be expected to go away on its own. OHSS occurs in about 1% of all cycles stimulated with ovulation-inducing drugs.

Another cause of infertility is the woman's own excess production of the hormone prolactin, which can be treated with bromocriptine or cabergoline, oral medications.

Intrauterine Insemination

Sometimes a couple's infertility is treated by artificially inseminating the woman with sperm from the male partner or from a donor. Intrauterine insemination (IUI) is a technique whereby sperm are injected directly into the woman's uterus, which allows them to bypass the cervical mucus. Therefore, this treatment is used when a woman has a cervical problem, when the man's sperm is less motile than normal, or when the man's sperm interacts poorly with the woman's cervical mucus. It's also a kind of "catchall" treatment that can be tried when doctors can't diagnose the cause of a couple's infertility.

Once IUI has taken place, the sperm must still swim into the woman's fallopian tubes, so this technique is not used when the woman's fallopian tubes are severely damaged or when the man's sperm is of poor quality. If a woman is in her early forties, she may also be advised against using her own eggs, because of the risk of birth defects as well as the difficulties of fertilization.

IUI usually begins by making sure that the woman's fallopian tubes are open, by means of either a hysterosalpingogram (HSG) or laparoscopy. An HSG involves introducing a special dye into the cervix so that it fills the uterus and fallopian tubes. The doctor can use an X ray to track the dye and thus gain valuable information about the size and shape of the uterus, as well as to see whether anything is blocking the fallopian tubes. A laparoscopy is a minor surgical procedure performed under general anesthesia in which the doctor inserts instruments through an incision in the woman's abdomen in order to view the woman's reproductive organs directly.

The next step in IUI is for the man to masturbate, so that his semen can be collected in a sterile container. The sample then undergoes sperm washing, a treatment that removes all the components from the semen except the sperm. Next, a speculum is inserted into the woman's vagina, and a catheter is inserted within the speculum into the woman's uterus. The sperm sample can be deposited through the catheter either into the woman's cervix or into her uterus. The entire procedure takes only a few minutes, and most women describe it as equal in discomfort to having a Pap smear done. As with a Pap smear, the woman may have some minor cramping.

If a woman is not taking any of the ovulation-inducing drugs described above, IUI is timed to take place just before she ovulates, as the sperm can live in her reproductive tract for a few days. The woman can have intercourse before or after the procedure without affecting the possibility of pregnancy. However, the success rate of IUI without drugs is lower than the success rate with drugs. If IUI is not successful after a few "unstimulated cycles"—cycles without drugs—then the woman may be given fertility drugs, such as Clomid and gonadotropins. The drugs increase the procedure's chance of success by increasing the number of eggs available to be fertilized.

Surgical Treatments for Women

As was just described, a laparoscopy is a procedure that allows a doctor to view a woman's lower abdomen. The doctor may then diagnose various conditions that might be causing the woman's infertility. In many cases, the doctor can treat these conditions at the same time, simply by inserting additional instruments through the laparoscope or through another small incision in the woman's lower abdomen.

Another surgical procedure, hysteroscopy, involves a viewing instrument known as a hysteroscope, which is inserted directly into a woman's vagina and cervix and on into the uterus. This procedure is used to diagnose particular uterine problems that may be causing infertility.

Both procedures may diagnose conditions for which there is not yet a treatment. In that case, the woman, her doctor, and possibly her partner may go on to choose a more complicated fertility treatment.

Reversals of Tubal Ligations and Vasectomies

Female sterilization involves tubal ligation, a sealing of the fallopian tubes, either by tying them off or by using a clip, band, or electric current. The latter procedure is one of the hardest to reverse. However, tubal ligation reversal has become far more successful in recent years, depending on the woman's age, the type of tubal ligation she had, and the length of the fallopian tubes left. Some 50% to 80% of all women who reverse this operation will eventually become pregnant, although they have a slightly higher risk of ectopic pregnancy.

The parallel sterilization procedure in men is known as a vasectomy, in which a tiny portion of the vas deferens on each side of the scrotum is removed and the two ends of the vas are sealed with sutures, clips, or electrical current. A vasectomy may be reversed if the severed ends of the vas deferens can be reconnected. Microsurgery, using very fine needles and suturing materials, has had some success with reversing vasectomies. However, a "successful" reversal—meaning that sperm is now present in the man's semen—does not necessarily ensure that the man will be able to father a child.

In Vitro Fertilization (IVF)

"In vitro" is Latin for "in the glass." The term refers to procedures that are done outside a living body—in the "glass" of test tubes, Petri dishes, or other laboratory containers. Specifically, in vitro fertilization is the fertilization of an egg and a sperm in a laboratory dish. (Although the popular term for a child conceived through IVF is "test-tube baby," the procedure acutally uses a small glass saucer.) If the fertilization is successful, the fertilized egg is transferred into a woman's uterus. Ideally, it will implant itself in the uterine wall and grow into a living fetus.

IVF was first developed for women who had problems with their fallopian tubes. Today, IVF is also used to treat female infertility caused by endometriosis and imbalances in the woman's immune system; for some types of male infertility; and in many cases of unexplained infertility.

Different clinics perform IVF differently, but the basic steps are as follows:

1. **Controlled Ovarian Hyperstimulation (COH).** COH stimulates the woman's ovaries to produce many eggs at once. The goal in IVF is to create embryos that can be successfully implanted into the woman's uterus and come to term. The more eggs there are to work with, the greater the chances that a healthy embryo will eventually be implanted. IVF is sometimes performed without COH, but doctors and patients usually prefer to increase their chances for success by increasing the number of available eggs. Therefore, to stimulate egg production, the woman is usually given an GnRH analog. This medication is chemically similar to the body's own natural GnRH, the gonadotropin-releasing hormone that stimulates the ovaries to release one egg each month. However, the analog suppresses women's natural hormonal responses, allowing her ovaries to respond more effectively to the extra stimulation of the artifical hormone.

2. **Egg Retrieval.** Vaginal ultrasound is used to find out how many eggs are in the woman's ovaries. Then the woman is given a local anesthetic and an ultrasound probe is inserted into her vagina. The doctor guides a needle through the vaginal wall and into the follicles. He or she then suctions or aspirates the eggs out of the follicles and into the needle. Another form of egg retrieval is laparoscopy (see above). In this case, eggs are retrieved through the laparoscope via a long,

thin needle inserted through the abdominal wall and into the follicles. This procedure requires general anesthesia.

3. **Fertilization of the Eggs and Cultivation of the Embryos.** Once the eggs are retrieved, they're evaluated for maturity. Only mature eggs should be fertilized, so insemination might take place within minutes, hours, or days after the eggs have been retrieved.

   On the day of retrieval, the male partner masturbates to produce semen. Sperm washing (see above) is conducted so that only the most motile sperm will be used. Then some sperm are put into each laboratory dish containing an egg, along with a growth medium, a substance that will allow the fertilized eggs to grow. The dishes are put into an incubator to keep them at the temperature of a woman's body. If successful, fertilization takes place within 16 to 18 hours. If the process continues to be successful, each embryo will divide into two cells about 12 hours after fertilization. The embryos will ideally continue to divide over the next two to five days, when they are ready to be transferred into the woman's uterus.

4. **Embryo Transfer.** Performed without anesthesia, this process takes less than half an hour. It involves suspending one or more embryos in a drop of culture medium and drawing them into a transfer catheter, a long, thin tube with a syringe at one end. The catheter is then inserted into the cervix and the syringe injects the embryos into the woman's uterus. Again, doctors and patients face a decision about how many embryos to transfer. Transferring more embryos offers a greater chance that at least one will implant in the woman's uterus, resulting in a pregnancy; but it also increases the risk of multiple births. Transferring fewer embryos lowers the chance of multiple pregnancy, but it also lowers the chance of getting pregnant. Doctors continue to debate the ideal number of embryos that should be implanted in an IVF procedure. Couples may decide to freeze, or cryopreserve, additional embryos, which can be thawed and transferred later on.

There are also several variations on IVF, all of which begin with stimulating and retrieving several eggs from the woman's ovaries and preparing the man's semen sample with sperm washing:

- **Gamete Intrafallopian Transfer (GIFT).** In GIFT, the eggs and sperm are inserted not into a laboratory dish but into the woman's fallopian tubes, as part of the procedure of egg retrieval. If GIFT is successful, an egg will be fertilized in the fallopian tubes, just as in natural reproduction. Ideally, the fertilized egg then travels into the uterus and implants there.
- **Zygote Intrafallopian Transfer (ZIFT);** also known as Pronuclear Stage Transfer (PROST). A zygote, or pronucleus, is an egg that has

been fertilized but has not yet undergone cell division. In ZIFT/PROST, eggs are retrieved as in IVF and fertilized in a laboratory dish as in IVF. But instead of growing in the dish for two to five days, they are transferred back into the woman's fallopian tubes the next day. Laparoscopy is used to make this second transfer. Again, the hope is that the fertilized eggs will divide and grow naturally and will travel into the woman's uterus and implant.

- **Tubal Embryo Transfer (TET).** In TET, eggs are transferred at a more mature stage than in GIFT or ZIFT/PROST, but at a less mature stage than in IVF. About 24 hours after eggs are fertilized (in the lab dish, as in IVF), when the embryos have reached the four- to eight-cell stage of division, they are transferred into the woman's fallopian tube. Once again, the hope is that the embryo will travel into the woman's uterus and implant there.

- **Assisted Hatching.** After eggs have been fertilized through IVF, assisted hatching may be used to improve the chances of the embryo actually implanting in the uterine wall. A microscopic hole is made in the zona pellucida (the "clear zone" surrounding the egg), to make it easier for an embryo to be released from the egg membrane. Either a miscrosurgical needle or chemicals may be used to make the hole.

Micromanipulation and Microsurgery for Male Infertility

The techniques discussed so far are used when, for whatever reason, a woman has trouble conceiving normally. Scientists have also developed techniques to respond to male infertility, particularly when the cause is a low sperm count or low sperm motility. Micromanipulation and microsurgery techniques can be used to ensure that a sperm fertilizes an egg or to retrieve sperm from an obstructed male genital tract. The following techniques are in various stages of development, and new developments are taking place even as this book is going to press.

These techniques are generally used in conjunction with IVF or other technologies. Virtually all are used after a woman has undergone COH to create extra eggs for the fertility speciality to work with:

- **Intracytoplasmic Sperm Injection (ICSI).** Once eggs are available outside the woman's body, the doctor uses a microsurgical needle to inject one sperm directly into an egg. Before this technique existed, a man was considered infertile if he had a low sperm count. Now, a man can be fertile if he can produce even a single sperm—as long as his female partner's eggs can be harvested.

- **Microinsemination.** The chances of fertilization are increased by concentrating sperm into a small drop of fluid and then placing it around the eggs. Again, this takes place in a lab dish, after the woman's eggs have been harvested, usually with the assistance of COH.

- **Testicular Sperm Extraction (TESE).** In this procedure, immature sperm cells are collected directly from the testes. Because these sperm cells are not fully mature, they would not normally be able to fertilize an egg. Scientists are exploring possibilities for using this genetic material to somehow fertilize a mature egg.

- **Round Spermatid Nuclear Injection (ROSNI).** In this procedure, TESE is followed by ICSI: the nucleus of an immature sperm cell (a round spermatid) is collected via TESE and then injected into an egg with ICSI. A few pregnancies have actually been achieved with this technique, which may be useful for infertility caused by azoospermia that cannot be corrected by surgery.

- **Microsurgical Epididymal Sperm Aspiration (MESA).** The epididymis is the organ where sperm cells are stored and where they mature. In this technique, microsurgery is used to collect sperm directly from the epididymis, an option that holds promise for men with obstruction of the vas deferens that cannot be corrected with surgery. A doctor makes a tiny opening through the scrotum and enters the epididymis, with the help of a microscope to avoid scarring the tissue inside the epididymis. Fluid is collected from the epididymis and examined microscopically to detect the presence of viable sperm. This procedure may require checking several sites within the epididymis, until live, moving sperm are finally located. The sperm collected in this manner can then be used in IVF, GIFT, or ZIFT/PROST.

- **Electroejaculation.** If a man has problems with ejaculation, this method of sperm collection may be in order. A probe is inserted into the man's rectum so that a low electrical voltage passes through the nerves that stimulate ejaculation. When semen has been collected, it is examined for viable sperm, which can then be used in one of the in vitro procedures described above.

Reproductive Technology Involving Donors

Many reproductive techniques involve the help of people who do not themselves wish to raise a child. Outsiders may donate sperm, eggs, or embryos. There have been cases in which a donated sperm and egg were implanted into a surrogate, who carried the pregnancy and gave birth to a child that was then given to two other people to raise.

- **Therapeutic Donor Insemination (TDI).** If a couple's infertility is traceable to the man, they may choose to have IUI with donated sperm.

Couples also choose this option when the male partner is known to have a hereditary or genetic disorder, such as hemophilia, Tay-Sachs disease, Huntington's chorea, or chromosomal abnormalities. Single women and lesbian couples may also choose this option. The sperm may come from an anonymous donor to a sperm bank or from a donor known to the parent(s).

• **Donor Oocytes (Egg Donation).** Some women are not able to produce enough healthy eggs of their own to undergo IVF, GIFT, or ZIFT/PROST. These women may use donor oocytes (eggs before ovulation). Women with abnormalities of the uterus are not candidates for this procedure. However, it has been used with success by women who were born without ovaries, have had their ovaries surgically removed, have experienced premature menopause, or have undergone chemotherapy or radiation therapy. In recent years, women of advanced age have also chosen to use donor eggs, to avoid chromosomal problems and to facilitate fertilization. The oocyte donor undergoes COH for two or three weeks and is then giving a shot of human chorionic gonadotropin (hCG) to trigger ovulation. About 24 hours later, the eggs are aspirated from her ovaries, evaluated for maturity, and fertilized in vitro by one of the procedures described above. Meanwhile, the recipient is also given GnRH analogs to suppress her own menstrual cycle and synchronize her timing with the donor. The recipient is also given hormones to encourage her uterine lining to thicken in preparation for pregnancy, as she must be ready to receive the eggs within a few days after retrieval. The embryos that result from the IVF procedure are then transferred to her uterus, where she carries them to term.

• **Surrogate Gestation (Surrogate Motherhood).** In one form of surrogacy, a woman carries a pregnancy that was created through a fertilized egg that is not her own; the resulting embryo is then implanted into her womb. In another form of surrogacy, IUI is used to implant the surrogate with a man's sperm, but the surrogate provides one of her own eggs.

THE HISTORY OF REPRODUCTIVE RIGHTS AND TECHNOLOGY

BEFORE 1960

Folk Practices and Traditional Medicine

From the earliest cultures that we know about, human beings have wondered about how to control conception, pregnancy, and birth. Fertility goddesses, midwives, folk wisdom, herbal remedies, and a range of medical traditions from around the globe have all been invoked as ways of preventing unwanted conceptions and engendering wanted pregnancies and births.

For centuries, infanticide—the killing of newborn babies—was probably the most widely used method of population control, given that techniques for either preventing conception or terminating pregnancies were unreliable. The early Greek philosophers Plato and Aristotle both recommended infanticide as a way of encouraging the "fit" and discouraging the "unfit."

Birth-control historian Linda Gordon suggests that infanticide was discarded as a widespread practice only when more reliable methods of contraception and abortion were discovered. Indeed, U.S. newspapers and trial transcripts suggest how frequently this method of population control was used in the eighteenth and nineteenth centuries.

Meanwhile, throughout many cultures, women also sought abortions, traditionally through the use of an abortifacient—a potion or compound that induced or was believed to induce abortion. German folk medicine recommended an herbal tea made of marjoram, thyme, parsley, and lavender, while both German and French women employed the root of worm fern. Until *Roe v. Wade* made abortion legal in the United States in 1973, U.S. women used a variety of "home remedies," including turpentine, castor oil, tansy tea, quinine water with a rusty nail soaked in it, horseradish, ginger, epsom salts, ammonia, mustard, gin with iron filings, rosemary, lavender, and opium. Many Latin American women continue to use herbal methods of abortion. (Of course, no one should try these methods without proper medical supervision; besides being far less effective than modern means of abortion, they could have potentially deadly side effects.)

Women have also tried to bring on abortions by such methods as exercise, heavy lifting, climbing trees, hot baths, jumping, and shaking. An ancient tradition that goes back to an eighth-century Sanskrit source—sitting over a pot of steam—was apparently used as late as the twentieth century by immigrant women on the Lower East Side of New York City (who sometimes used the steam from a pot of stewed onions).

In addition, women have tried aborting their own pregnancies, inserting such objects as wire coat hangers into their vaginas. Clearly, such means are enormously risky and painful, and women often died of hemorrhage (excessive bleeding), infection, or other complications. Women using any of these methods—abortifacients, activity, or self-abortion—might also risk permanent harm to their reproductive systems as well as illness and death.

Birth Control and Abortion in Nineteenth-Century America

Until the middle of the nineteenth century, both Protestant and Catholic traditions held that abortion before "quickening" (the mother's experience of the fetus moving, usually during the fourth or fifth month of pregnancy) was not a crime. Both U.S. and British common law took this view as well. (Common law is the unwritten legal tradition that both the British and early

U.S. systems considered to be in effect until superseded by a written law.) Evidence from women's diaries and letters also suggests that prequickening abortion was both commonplace and widely accepted throughout the eighteenth and nineteenth centuries.

During the nineteenth century, legal opinion began to turn against abortion. The first U.S. statute against abortion was enacted in Connecticut in 1821. By 1841, 10 of the 26 U.S. states had made abortion a crime as part of routine revisions of legal codes.

Medical opinion was changing, too, as women's health passed out of the care of largely female folk healers and midwives and into the hands of mostly male professionally trained physicians. The American Medical Association (AMA) began to investigate abortions in 1857 under the leadership of Horatio B. Storer, a Harvard-trained doctor who sought to criminalize all induced abortions. In 1866 and 1867, Storer published books directed at women and men, respectively, to convince them that life began not at quickening but at conception and that therefore abortion was murder.

Religious opinion seemed to follow suit. In 1869, Pope Pius IX announced that, in the view of the Roman Catholic Church, all abortion was murder. Early U.S. feminists, including Elizabeth Cady Stanton, also tended to see abortion as "the degradation of women," as Stanton wrote in the first volume of *Revolution*, a suffragist journal. (Suffragists fought for women's right to vote.)

Yet U.S. abortionists continued to practice, and if their cases came to trial, they were often acquitted. In a series of articles that ran in 1870 and 1871, the *New York Times* estimated that there were some 200 full-time abortionists in New York City. Abortion was probably safer for women than childbirth. Even today, far more women die in childbirth (1 in 13,000) than from early-term abortions (0.04 in 100,000).

Then, in 1873, Congress passed the Comstock Law, striking a major blow against both abortion and contraception. The Comstock Law explicitly defined as obscene all contraceptive devices and all information about contraception. It became a federal crime to send any such information or equipment through the U.S. mail.

The force behind the Comstock Law was Anthony Comstock, head of the New York Society for the Suppression of Vice. Comstock was also instrumental in the passage of anticontraception laws in 22 states. The strictest such laws were passed in Connecticut and Massachusetts.

Comstock did not just work on a legislative level; he had been named a special federal agent charged with preventing the distribution and use of "obscene" items. His work took place in a climate when even feminists and suffragists continued to oppose birth control, advocating celibacy and abstinence rather than mechanical means of preventing pregnancy. At the same time, government and economic leaders urged population growth to fill the new farming territories to the West and the new factories in the East. In 1905, for example, President Theodore Roosevelt denounced birth control and said that the trend toward smaller families was a sign of moral disease.

Science and Pseudoscience

Over the centuries, in England and northern Europe, a scientific approach to human reproduction was developing alongside of folk and religious traditions. In the 1670s, Dutch scientist Antonie von Leeuwenhoek first saw sperm under a microscope, while in 1790, the first child conceived through artificial insemination was born.

Artificial insemination techniques continued to fascinate scientists. In 1884, a wealthy Philadelphia couple trying to have a child approached Dr. William Pancoast, a professor of medicine. Pancoast put the wife under anesthesia, found the handsomest medical student in his class, and used the young man's sperm to impregnate the wife, unbeknownst to either the woman or her husband. Eventually, Pancoast saw that the child resembled his biological father, and so he confessed to the adoptive father what he had done. The man asked only that his wife never be told the truth.

Even as government and industrial leaders were calling for increased population, a kind of science called eugenics warned that the population was increasing too quickly, with the "wrong kind" of person. Today, eugenics is no longer considered reputable science, but in the late nineteenth and early twentieth centuries, many medical professionals and researchers thought that Charles Darwin's theory of evolution, often called—somewhat inaccurately—"survival of the fittest," had a direct application to their own society. If the "unfit" had too many children and the "fit" had not enough, eugenicists believed, society would soon decline. Today's scientists believe that evolution does not work nearly so quickly nor so simply, but eugenics appealed to a society with a mostly northern and western European background facing a sudden influx of immigrants from southern and eastern Europe and a migration of African Americans from south to north. To many scientists of the time, Italians, Irish, Greeks, Poles, Russians, and Africans were clearly "inferior races" whose propagation had to be stopped.

In 1910, therefore, the Eugenics Record Office was established in Cold Spring Harbor, New York, with the purpose of training field workers to gather family histories throughout the United States. This knowledge, eugenicists believed, could encourage the breeding of "good" families while discouraging the breeding of "bad" ones. In 1914, pioneer eugenicist Harry Laughlin, head of that office, published a Model Eugenical Sterilization Law proposing sterilization of the "socially inadequate"—that is, people supported in institutions for the "feebleminded, insane, criminalistic, epileptic, inebriate [drunken], diseased, blind, deaf, deformed; and dependent," including "orphans, ne'er-do-wells, tramps, the homeless, and paupers." Indiana had already passed a law allowing sterilization on eugenic grounds, with Connecticut following suit soon after. By the time the model law was published, they had been joined by 10 other states.

Amid the very immigrants that the eugenicists feared worked a young woman named Margaret Sanger. When Sanger tried to help a doctor save the life of tenement dweller Sadie Sachs from the effects of a self-induced abortion, she realized that the working women and housewives of New York's immigrant neighborhoods were in dire need of contraception. These families, Sanger believed, would be condemned to poverty, and the women doomed to exhaustion and early death, if women could not choose how many children they wished to have. Sanger coined the phrase *birth control* and made up her mind to work against the Comstock laws.

In 1914, Sanger began to publish *The Woman Rebel*, a feminist monthly magazine explaining the birth control techniques she had learned about in France. In 1916, she opened the nation's first birth control clinic in the Brownsville section of Brooklyn, New York. Hundreds of women came to find out how they could control their own reproductive abilities—but within a month Sanger was arrested, along with her sister and a friend. Police closed the clinic, making it clear to Sanger that she had to turn to the legislature so that birth control could become legal and widely available.

Contraception and Forced Sterilization

The society in which Sanger lived had not yet allowed women the right to vote. In addition, deep conflicts existed about acknowledging women's sexuality, and very different expectations existed for different classes. Most of society's middle and upper classes—including most suffragists—saw women as virtuously asexual, a civilizing influence on men, who were viewed as sexual predators, sinful and out of control. If women could not stop men's sexual overtures, according to this view, all of civilization would revert to barbarism. To acknowledge that women were sexual creatures was tantamount to giving in to evil.

The only women who were sexual, in the eyes of many middle- and upper-class citizens, were working women, immigrants, and African Americans. The women of those "races" and classes were seen as little better than prostitutes by those who dominated the society. In this climate, it was very difficult to overturn the Comstock laws—and indeed, birth control continued to be illegal despite repeated legislative efforts. In Connecticut, for example, contraception remained against the law until the landmark 1965 Supreme Court case of *Griswold v. Connecticut.*

Meanwhile, Sanger went on to found the American Birth Control League in 1921. She chose the strategy of appealing to doctors for support, suggesting that they, and not the government, should decide what contraception they might prescribe to their patients.

At the same time, the eugenics movement and the fear of the "lower orders" continued unabated. By 1924, some 3,000 U.S. residents had been forcibly sterilized, most (2,500) in California. The same year, Virginia passed a Eugenical Sterilization Act based on Laughlin's model law. Virginia saw its efforts to prevent reproduction of the "unfit" as a way to relieve the state's tax burden, for by then Virginia supported several public facilities for the "insane" and "feebleminded." The Virginia law also protected doctors who performed sterilizations from being sued for malpractice. "Heredity plays an important part in the transmission of insanity, idiocy, imbecility, epilepsy, and crime . . . " stated the law, and "defective persons" were a "menace to society."

Carrie Buck, a 17-year-old unwed mother, was the first person to be sterilized under the Virginia law. Carrie was examined by sociologist Arthur Estabrook, of the Eugenics Record Office, who along with a Red Cross nurse testified that Carrie's baby, Vivian, was "below average" and "not quite normal." Carrie's mother, Emma, had also been institutionalized, and the superintendent of the facility where Emma was held testified that she had "a record of immorality, prostitution, untruthfulness and syphilis." The Buck family in general, the superintendent said, belonged "to the shiftless, ignorant, and worthless class of anti-social whites of the South."

Carrie Buck's sterilization was finally authorized in the 1927 Supreme Court case, *Buck v. Bell*. Justice Oliver Wendell Holmes wrote the opinion authorizing Buck's sterilization, finding that "It is better for all the world if, instead of waiting to execute degenerate offspring for crime, or to let them starve for their imbecility, society can prevent those who are manifestly unfit from continuing their kind . . . "

Some 60 years later, historian Paul Lombardo discovered that Carrie Buck was of normal intelligence, as was her daughter, Vivian, who went on to become a solid B student at the local school. Vivian's birth was not even the result of Carrie's sexual activity, but rather of her rape by a relative of the family with whom she had lived.

From the 1920s through the 1950s, these two contradictory trends continued. On the one hand, women and men were effectively forbidden access to safe, legal contraception. Abortion was either an illegal procedure or one that very few women had access to, usually on the grounds that it was an operation that they needed to save their lives.

Yet at the same time, people were being forcibly sterilized by laws that considered them "unfit" to reproduce. A 1935 Oklahoma law calling for the forced sterilization of repeat criminals was the subject of another Supreme Court case, which was heard in 1942. Justice William O. Douglas, writing the majority opinion in *Skinner v. Oklahoma*, struck down the Oklahoma law—yet at the time, some 13 states had laws calling for the sterilization of criminals. Although the Skinner case set an important precedent, it did not overturn *Buck v. Bell*. To this day, there is no Supreme Court decision to overrule a law allowing for the sterilization of the "feebleminded."

Another trend continued throughout the 1930s and 1940s, though at the time it was barely noticeable: Scientists continued to discover new ways to promote reproduction. In 1937, for example, the *New England Journal of Medicine*, perhaps the most prestigious medical magazine in the United States, published an editorial entitled "Conception in a Watch Glass," proposing the notion of in vitro fertilization. The following year, scientists recorded the first survival of sperm after freezing. These technologies would explode several decades later, but at that point, they were just daring ideas discussed by a few farsighted scientists.

THE 1960s

The Pill and the Griswold Case

By 1960, contraception was legal in many states—though still not in Connecticut. In that year, reproductive technology took a dramatic new turn with the invention of "the Pill," an oral contraceptive that relied on hormones to prevent pregnancy.

Previously, contraceptive devices included various versions of the condom and the diaphragm—actual barriers that would prevent semen from entering a woman's uterus. Both the condom and the diaphragm had to be either put on or inserted; and both might fail while being used. The Pill, on the other hand, had close to a 100% success rate, and all that was needed was for a woman to remember to take it every morning—she didn't need to stop at the height of passion, convince a man to wear it, nor even admit to her male partner that she had thought to bring a birth control device with her.

In the minds of many, the Pill introduced a sexual revolution into U.S. society, enabling women and their male partners to enjoy sex without the prospect of procreation for the first time in human history. Women's sexual lives, especially, were changed when the possibility of pregnancy was completely within their control.

Legal changes followed the social transformation. In 1965, a landmark Supreme Court case, *Griswold v. Connecticut*, established that the birth control clinic opened by Dr. C. Lee Buxton and Estelle Griswold in 1961 was indeed legal. Buxton and Griswold had been arrested and fined for providing birth control to married couples, but the Planned Parenthood Federation—the descendant of Margaret Sanger's American Birth Control League—took their case to court. The Supreme Court ruled that married couples had the right to privacy, which included the right to use contraception. Two years later, President Lyndon Baines Johnson approved a $20 million annual budget for family planning services, signaling a new public acceptance of contraception, at least for married couples.

Changing Attitudes Toward Abortion

When the 1960s began, abortion was considered a crime by most people—and all state legislatures. Gradually, though, legal and medical experts begin to push for reform of abortion laws to allow the procedure when the woman's life or health was in danger, when the child would be born with severe defects, or when the pregnancy resulted from rape or incest. Although feminists and doctors had vehemently opposed abortion a century earlier, the American Medical Association and the National Organization for Women (NOW) came out in favor of legalized abortion in 1967 and 1968, respectively. Also in 1968, the National Association for the Repeal of Abortion Laws (NARAL) was founded.

Yet some attitudes were changing in the opposite direction. The Roman Catholic Church maintained its position on abortion while also declaring, in Pope Paul VI's *Humanae Vitae* (1968), that oral contraceptives and all other "artificial" means of birth control were contrary to the teachings of the church. The following year, the American Civil Liberties Union (1969), Planned Parenthood, and the World Population Organization all came out in favor of legalizing abortion.

Reproductive Technology Moves Forward

Although most Americans were barely aware of the growing field of reproductive technology, scientists were continuing to study human reproduction, often with astonishing results. In 1969, the pioneering embryologist Robert Edwards wrote an article in *Nature* magazine about the possibility of artificially fertilizing human eggs.

THE 1970S

The End of the Comstock Law

The Comstock law—which banned novels and other literature deemed obscene as well as scientific information—had been under attack for many years. In 1971, Congress deleted the portions of the law that applied to contraception and abortion. The following year, in *Eisenstadt v. Baird*, the Supreme Court struck down a Massachusetts law forbidding the sale and distribution of contraception to unmarried people. The same right of privacy that had obtained in *Griswold*, ruled the Court, extended to all people, married or not.

Abortion and Antiabortion

The early 1970s saw activity in both directions regarding abortion rights. Alaska, Hawaii, and New York all repealed their antiabortion laws in 1970, with New York's feminist-led campaign being viewed as a national model for other states.

Partially in response, two new antiabortion groups were formed in 1971. Both groups called upon the notion of antiabortion activists being "pro-life": Pro-lifers for Survival, an antinuclear group (responding to the generally "pro-choice" atmosphere of the rest of the antinuclear movement); and Feminists for Life (responding to the pro-choice consensus that prevailed among most feminists). (As antiabortion activists called themselves "pro-life," so did feminists develop the term "pro-choice.")

By 1972, 14 states had passed laws allowing for "therapeutic" abortion—abortion deemed necessary to preserve the woman's life or health. Thus, if a woman in those states could find a doctor to say that an abortion was necessary to her mental health, she might be allowed to have the procedure. Women without money or connections, however, might have a far more difficult time finding the "right" doctor.

Then, on January 22, 1973, the Supreme Court transformed the legal, social, and political climate in the United States by handing down *Roe v. Wade*, a 7–2 decision that the right to privacy established in *Griswold* and *Eisenstadt* extended to women's right to choose an abortion. *Roe* specified that states could regulate abortion in particular ways: to protect women's health starting in the second trimester, and to protect "the potential life of the fetus" during the third trimester. (States might even prohibit third-trimester abortions for the fetus's sake.) During the first trimester, however, a woman's right to an abortion was absolute. And during the second trimester, a woman's health was the only basis on which the procedure might be restricted.

As a result of *Roe*, all state laws outlawing early abortion were struck down. Also as a result of *Roe*, the antiabortion movement—now known as "pro-life"—became a national force. This movement had existed for some years: Dr. Jack Willke and his wife had founded "Right to Life of Greater Cincinnati" in 1970, for example, the first and largest local right-to-life group in the United States. But the powerful nationwide movement whose long-term goal was to abolish abortion and whose short-term goal was to restrict it, was a direct result of *Roe v. Wade*. Thus in 1973, Willke and his wife established the National Right to Life Committee, a group that would eventually include some 10 million members and would become the largest national pro-life organization.

Reproductive Technology and Legal Disputes

Even as pro-choice and pro-life movements were forming around *Roe*, developments in reproductive technology were creating new legal, medical, and social questions. In 1972, Vanderbilt University Professor Dr. Pierre Soupart became the first U.S. scientist to fertilize an egg in vitro. Soupart went on to apply for a government grant to study the safety of IVF techniques, but he died in 1981 before receiving his funding.

Yet lack of study did not stop doctors from offering the new techniques to their patients. In 1973, Doris and John Del Zio became the first U.S. couple to try the IVF procedure that Soupart had demonstrated only the year before. This speedy adoption of unproven technology would continue to characterize U.S. fertility medicine. From the very beginning, reproductive innovations were tried out on individual female patients before they had been extensively tested on lab animals, let alone studied in controlled human experiments. IVF was performed on humans in 1973, and the first IVF baby was successfully born in 1978. Yet the first successful IVF baboon was not born until 1979.

In fact, the Del Zios' procedure was interrupted by the outraged supervisor of one of the physicians involved in the treatment, putting a halt to the experimental effort. Eventually, the Del Zios brought a lawsuit, claiming that Doris's only chance to become a mother had been sabotaged by the supervisor's interference.

Abortion and Forced Sterilization

The 1970s continued to be marked by increasingly contradictory developments. On the one hand, abortion rights activists celebrated the expanded freedom and choice that they saw as part of women's new right to choose abortion. The number of legal abortions shot up quickly after *Roe*, so that by decade's end, the rate was roughly 1.5 million per year (today the rate is almost as high: about 1.2 million legal abortions per year). Feminists and abortion rights activists cheered at the thought that unsafe "back-alley" abortions were a thing of the past; that women could choose sexual activity with men without also choosing pregnancy; and that women's expanded role in the economic and political arenas was supported by their right to make their own decisions about childbearing and pregnancy.

Pro-life activists saw abortion as little more than legalized murder, and they were appalled both by the number of abortions and by the procedure's apparently widespread acceptance. These activists had a variety of views, but many of them approached the world from a religious perspective—their ranks included large numbers of Catholics and fundamentalist Protestants—and they tended to see abortion both as a sin in itself and as a sign that women were rejecting their God-given role as a nurturing, maternal influence on society. Many pro-life activists objected to the idea that women should be sexually free outside of marriage, or that sex should be viewed as an end in itself rather than as part of the creation of a family.

In addition, many pro-life activists were disturbed by what they saw as the commercialization of U.S. culture, an alienated and impersonal focus on money and material things that seemed to them to extend even into the doctor-patient relationship. Thus, they accused doctors who performed abortions of operating "abortion mills" largely for profit, at the expense of women who would not have chosen such a brutal and psychologically damaging procedure had they not been manipulated by money-hungry doctors. In decades to come, these activists would also be concerned about the way that human bodies seemed to be divided into parts and functions, all of which were for sale or rent—egg, sperm, womb. Where once there had been nurturing family relationships, these activists argued, now there were commercial transactions, creating a world in which parents failed to care for their children while sexual partners exploited each other without consequence. This larger world-view shaped both the rhetoric and the intensity of much of the pro-life movement.

Meanwhile, another sphere was attracting the attention of pro-choice feminists. Forced sterilization—a legacy of the eugenics movement—continued apace in the 1970s, particularly among Native Americans, African Americans, Puerto Rican Americans and women on welfare. While some feminists, at least, saw both abortion and forced sterilization as reproductive rights issues, the pro-life movement generally ignored the claims of women of color and welfare rights activists that large numbers of women were being coerced into sterilization.

It is difficult to obtain comprehensive statistics on Native American women's experience with the Indian Health Service (IHS), the major form of health care for Indian women. But figures collected by Congress's General Accounting Office (GAO) at the request of South Dakota senator James Abourezk between 1973 and 1976 are suggestive. Although the GAO studied only four of the 12 regions covered by the IHS, they found that at least 3,406 Indian women had been sterilized in those regions over 46 months.

Given that in all of the United States, there were only 100,000 Native American women of childbearing age, the fact that 3.4% of them had been sterilized in four years indicates that a significant percentage of Indian women were being stripped of their ability to have children. In the IHS's Oklahoma region, the figures are even higher: 1,761 of 17,000 Native American women of childbearing age were sterilized—more than 10%. Native Americans themselves claimed that 40% of Native women and 10% of Native men were sterilized during that decade.

Sterilization of Native American women was completely paid for by federal funds. These funds were also used to pay for the sterilization of non-Indian women on welfare. In 1970, the passage of the Family Planning Act led the Department of Health, Education, and Welfare (HEW; the old title of today's Department of Health and Human Services, or DHHS) to dramatically accelerate their sterilization programs. Thus, the rate of sterilization of all U.S. women jumped 350% over five years.

Again, the statistics are instructive. HEW records show that from 1907 through 1964, the average annual number of women sterilized was 63,000. Yet between 1970 and 1977, from 192,000 to 548,000 women were sterilized each year.

These efforts were only one aspect of the United States' international policy, according to a story published in the *St. Louis Dispatch*. Dr. R. T. Ravenholt, director of the U.S. Agency for International Development (USAID), was quoted there as saying that he hoped to sterilize 25% of the world's 570 million fertile women, as part of the "normal operation of U.S. commercial interests around the world."

An article by Beverly Horsburgh in the January 1996 *Cardozo Law Review* asserts that from 1970 to 1980, sterilization rates for U.S. women had tripled, particularly among women of color and women on welfare. To some extent, this reflected the liberalized indications for sterilization that the American College of Obstetricians and Gynecologists (ACOG) had developed in the 1970s. It may also have been the result of the forced or semi-coerced sterilization of women of color and women on welfare: As of 1982, according to Hosburgh, 15% of all white women had been sterilized, as compared to 24% of African American women, 35% of Puerto Rican women, and 42% of Native American women.

In 1977, the case of *Relf v. Weinberger* was brought against HEW Secretary Caspar Weinberger, alleging that welfare mothers had been threatened with the loss of their benefits if they did not agree to be sterilized. The welfare rights protestors won, and the case theoretically put an end to the forced sterilization of women on welfare. Yet activists continued to charge that welfare recipients were still being coerced into having "the operation," as tubal ligation was commonly called. Moreover, as in the case of Carrie

Buck, women in institutions for the mentally ill and mentally retarded continued to be sterilized into the mid-1970s.

Meanwhile, in 1977, right-to-life leader Illinois representative Henry Hyde sponsored the Hyde Amendment in Congress, making federal Medicaid funds for abortion unavailable (except in procedures needed to save the mother's life). Thus women on Medicaid could use federal funds to be sterilized but not to have an abortion.

THE 1980s

From Right-to-Life to Operation Rescue

During this decade, the Supreme Court decisions generally protected women's right to abortion and struck down laws that sought to limit that right. In two 1980 cases, the Court did permit both state and federal governments to refuse public funds for abortions, and in 1981 the Court ruled that states could require minors to get parental consent before obtaining an abortion. Yet for the most part, the Court said "no" to restrictions on abortion. States were not allowed to require women to wait 24 hours before obtaining abortions; they could not insist that doctors tell women about fetal development or show women pictures of developing fetuses; they could not require women to get consent for abortions from their husbands; and they could not require reports to be filed that included the names of doctors performing abortions. Even minors had to be given the chance to bypass their parents by taking their case to a judge.

Right-to-life groups were increasingly frustrated with these rulings, especially because, on the political level, they had won. The conservative right-to-life politician Ronald Reagan had been elected president in 1980, a victory that pro-life groups expected to usher in a new age of Christian and family values. The Religious Right/New Right groups that sprung up around Reagan were all strongly pro-life, as were the president's appointees to the Supreme Court and executive positions.

Yet the national consensus remained strongly pro-choice, and abortions continued to be available to women throughout the nation—at least, to women who did not depend upon public funding. To complicate matters, the long-established pro-life groups like the National Right to Life Committee found themselves at odds with the New Right groups that emerged in the late 1970s and early 1980s. Indeed, some observers believed that the New Right groups had been established precisely in order to woo pro-life support away from the old groups toward a new political agenda, an agenda far more pro-business and multi-issue than that of the first pro-life groups.

Moreover, even as Congress became more conservative on other issues, political support for choice grew stronger. According to a *New York*

Times/CBS report, 74% of the first-year members of Congress were pro-choice in 1982, up from only 54% in 1980. In 1983, pro-life Congressional leaders floated a proposed constitutional amendment seeking to overturn *Roe v. Wade* by asserting that abortion was not a right secured by the Constitution. Yet when the amendment was proposed to the Senate, it fell 18 votes short of the 2/3 majority that it needed. More and more, it seemed that the old-line right-to-life groups were failing to win the nation to their side.

As a result, a new kind of pro-life group began to emerge, one that relied less on legislative efforts and more on the direct-action tactics of militant protest and civil disobedience that many had associated with feminists and pro-choice groups. Operation Rescue was founded by Randall Terry in 1988, with the goal of keeping abortion clinics from operating and preventing individual women from obtaining abortions. Other groups with similar agendas sprung up on both the national and local levels.

The so-called rescue movement engaged in a technique known as "sidewalk counseling": protestors would surround a woman seeking to enter a clinic where abortions were provided, talking urgently to her and showing her pictures of fetuses. Sometimes the protestors went a step further and blockaded clinic entrances or parking lots; publicized the names of clinic staff; or protested outside the homes of doctors who worked at the clinics. Because abortion is generally not performed in a hospital, and because many hospitals had not wanted to be associated with abortion, health clinics had sprung up specializing in abortions (though most provided other services as well). Separated physically from other medical facilities and marginalized in the medical community, abortion clinics and staff were easier targets than the providers of other types of medical services.

As a result of Operation Rescue and similar groups, many doctors stopped providing abortions, and many clinics shut their doors. Combined with the loss of Medicaid funding for abortions, this meant that, throughout the 1980s, the availability of abortion services declined drastically. In many parts of the United States, women had to travel a considerable distance to locate a doctor or clinic who would provide them with an abortion: in 1986, 32% of women of childbearing age lived in counties that had no abortion providers. Once again, this was a particular hardship for low-income women, including many women of color.

Sperm Banks and Venture Capital

On the reproductive technology front, IVF procedures began to be used with increasing frequency during the 1980s. Sperm banks became big business, as did other fertility treatments. Venture capitalist Lawrence Suscy, for example, entered into a partnership with physicist and cattle breeder

Richard Seed, who hoped to adapt fertility techniques developed for cattle to use on human beings. Suscy planned to develop a national chain of fertility clinics, charging $4,000 to $7,000 per treatment, with some 30,000 to 50,000 women expected to apply. "Volume is nothing, margin is everything," Suscy told *Fortune* magazine.

Some observers were concerned that the number of fertility clinics was expanding without sufficient government regulation. In 1982, there were only a handful of fertility clinics in the United States; by 1985, there were 169. Yet about half of these could not claim a single successful live birth—a fact of which many patients remained unaware.

Still, fertility treatments continue to be developed and rushed onto the market. In 1984, Dr. Richard Marss announced the first U.S. birth of a child conceived from a frozen embryo. Soon, frozen embryos would become commonplace in U.S. fertility treatments: The embryos could be created in an IVF procedure and then stored indefinitely, to be thawed as needed. A woman might be impregnated with an embryo one year, and then later, when she was ready for a second child, be impregnated with another embryo that had been created at the same time as the first one. Critics warned that no one yet knew what effects freezing might have on an embryo—whether children created by this means would face medical problems later in life. Yet the demand for fertility services was so high—at least from a small, wealthy segment of the population—that doctors continued to performed the treatments as requested.

Why were couples so eager to try these new fertility treatments? In 1991, Pulitzer Prize–winning author Susan Faludi published *Backlash: The Undeclared War against American Women,* in which she suggests a reason. Faludi charged that throughout the 1980s, women were pressured to return to traditional roles of childrearing and made to feel both ashamed and anxious if they had chosen to spend their twenties and thirties focusing on career rather than family. Specifically, in 1982, the media had reported an alleged dramatic rise in women's infertility, which journalists attributed to women's delaying childbirth in favor of career. Yet, Faludi pointed out, the study on which the reporting was based had involved a group of French women married to infertile husbands who had all been trying to get pregnant using ART techniques. In fact, for women in their thirties and forties, fertility had risen since 1965.

Yet if Faludi's argument was correct, women were being led to believe that they were in grave danger of being childless. In such a climate, doctors offering new fertility treatments were highly sought-after—even if they had never actually helped patients have children.

Sterilization

Despite the new contraceptive techniques that were becoming available, many women continued to be sterilized. Throughout the 1980s, the rate of sterilization for African-American women continued to increase. In 1985, one clinic serving mostly African-American clients reported that 45% of black mothers chose tubal ligation after their first child had been born. Whether these women would have chosen another means of contraception under other circumstances—say, had funding or educational support for less permanent birth control been available; or had they not been subtly or overtly pressured by doctors or social workers—is a matter for speculation. What is clear is that in 1987, 24% of the entire U.S. population of child-bearing women had been sterilized. Even as the major media were warning "career women" of the dangers of delaying childbirth, women elsewhere in the economy were choosing or being influenced to choose sterility.

Ironically, in 1987, the federal government was providing 97% of the funding for sterilization, as opposed to less than 1% for abortions. Moreover, infertility procedures did not receive public funding, even though black families—who were more likely than white families to receive public funding—were also twice as likely to be infertile.

A 1984 court decision (*Oil, Chemical & Atomic Workers v. American Cyanamid Co.*) upheld the notion that women's infertility was a purely private matter rather than a public responsibility. Women working certain jobs at American Cynamid were required to show proof of sterility before being allowed to hold the jobs, as the company was aware that chemicals in the workplace might damage a fetus. The union brought suit, claiming that the corporation had no right to make sterility a condition of employment. The court found for the company, ruling that since women had the choice of either leaving their jobs or being sterilized, their rights were not being violated.

The "Webster" Decision: A New Direction for the Court

In 1989, the Supreme Court handed down another momentous decision that would have far-reaching consequences for reproductive rights. *Webster v. Reproductive Health Services* was a case arising from a 1986 Missouri law that was itself the result of a strong pro-life movement in that state. The Missouri law stated explicitly that life begins at conception. It banned the use of public funds for the purpose of counseling women who wanted to have abortions (except to save their lives), said that abortions could not be performed in public facilities (except to save a woman's life), and required doctors to test the fetuses of all women pregnant for 20 weeks or more who were seeking abortions to see if the fetuses were viable.

When *Webster* reached the High Court, the administration of President George H. W. Bush filed an *amicus* brief, asking the Court to overturn *Roe v. Wade*. On April 9, some half a million people marched on Washington in the March for Women's Equality/Women's Lives, the largest Washington demonstration since the Vietnam War. Numerous other protests accompanied the march, including 200,000 letters sent to Attorney General Dick Thornburgh, asking him to drop the administration's request to end *Roe*. A few weeks later, on April 26, the Court heard oral arguments, and it ruled on July 3.

Although the Court failed to overturn *Roe*, its decision in *Webster* distressed many pro-choice activists, for the Court upheld much of the Missouri law. Moreover, a sizeable number of Justices did vote to overturn *Roe*, leading many observers to believe that the Court would strike down *Roe* the next chance it got. (For details, see chapter 2).

In addition, *Webster* made it clear that the Court would look kindly on individual states passing restrictive antiabortion laws. Louisiana and Utah went on to ban virtually all abortions, hoping that their laws would become test cases that would lead the Court to overturn *Roe*. Other states instituted a number of restrictive measures, such as the mandatory waiting periods and "informed consent" provisions (requiring women to look at state-prepared materials or hear state-scripted lectures providing information about adoption) that had been overturned in earlier cases.

Despite the Court's action, a majority of the American people still came out strongly pro-choice. According to a Harris poll taken soon after the decision, almost 60% of Americans opposed *Webster* and supported *Roe*.

THE 1990s

Casey and Clinic Violence

In the final years of the Bush administration, federal policies on abortion continued to grow ever more restrictive, and the Supreme Court seemed more antiabortion than ever. In 1991, for example, the Supreme Court decided *Rust v. Sullivan* and *State of New York v. Sullivan*, two cases upholding a 1988 regulation of the Department of Health and Human Services (DHHS), which forbade staff at federally funded family planning clinics from counseling women about abortions, referring them to places where they might obtain abortions, or even informing women that abortion was a legal option (informally known as the "gag rule"). In 1992, the Court handed down *Planned Parenthood v. Casey*, in which it explicitly overturned many of its rulings of the 1980s. Suddenly, the Court would permit waiting periods, informed consent laws, and a whole host of other abortion restrictions that it had formerly deemed unconstitutional.

Yet the Court still failed to overturn *Roe*; indeed, in *Casey*, the Court explicitly upheld *Roe*, even though it offered a new definition for *Roe's* protections: Instead of viewing abortion as a fundamental right as *Roe* had seemed to do, the Court would now allow restrictions on abortion so long as they did not constitute an "undue burden" on a woman's ability to choose. (See chapter 2.)

Pro-choice activists greeted *Casey* with dismay, but many in the pro-life movement felt that the country was still very far from outlawing a procedure that they viewed as both immoral and destructive to society. Then liberal, pro-choice Bill Clinton was elected president in 1992, seeming to both sides to signal a new era. Both pro-choice and pro-life activists believed that having Clinton in the White House meant that pro-choice forces might now have the upper hand.

The most militant wing of the pro-life movement eventually responded with violence. In March 1993, Michael Griffin killed abortion provider Dr. David Gunn in front of a clinic in Pensacola, Florida, ushering in a new wave of violence at clinics and at the homes of abortion providers. By December 1994, clinic-related violence had doubled, resulting in the deaths of five people and the wounding of many more.

Traditional right-to-life leaders were appalled by this trend, as were some of the militant "rescue" groups. Some leaders, however, issued statements arguing that the true violence was taking place inside the clinics, and that any efforts to save the lives of the unborn were well worth the price of a few "murderers'" lives.

The federal government responded with a law called FACE, the Freedom of Access to Clinic Entrances, passed by Congress in May 1994, making it a federal crime to prevent either patients or staff from entering abortion clinics. Soon afterward, U.S. Attorney General Janet Reno assigned federal marshals to defend clinics around the country. In December 1994, the Justice Department organized a task force on the issue, working closely with a grand jury investigation into the possibility of a nationwide conspiracy. No evidence of a conspiracy was ever found.

Meanwhile, frightened for their lives, their families, and their reputations, many doctors stopped providing abortions, while many clinics shut their doors. In 1996, 86% of all U.S. counties had no abortion provider. In 1997, the Centers for Disease Control and Prevention released data showing that U.S. abortions had dropped to their lowest rate in 20 years: 1.3 million in 1993 and 1.2 million in 1994.

Even after clinic violence declined during the decade's second half, pro-choice activists were concerned that restrictions on abortion and the decline in abortion services meant that in practice, many U.S. women no longer had a choice, especially low-income women and teenagers. Moreover, activists worried that the various delays and obstacles built into the procedure in many states—the 24-hour waiting period, the informed consent provision, the lack of a facility in one's own county—were leading women to have abortions later and later. Earlier abortions are far safer medically, as well as less traumatic emotionally. Abortion rights activists feared that by making abortions harder to get, pro-life activists were also making abortion more dangerous.

Norplant and "The Shot"

Two new forms of contraception emerged in the early 1990s. In 1990, the FDA approved Norplant, a form of contraception that was surgically implanted, had to be surgically removed, and could remain in place for up to five years. In 1992, after a lengthy battle with such groups as the National Black Women's Health Project, the FDA gave the go-ahead to Depo-Provera, a hormonal contraceptive known as "the Shot" because it was administered through an injection.

Welfare rights groups, some feminists, and many women of color eventually objected to both Norplant and the Shot when welfare recipients began to be strongly advised—some said coerced—to make use of them. Although Norplant and the Shot are reversible, Norplant has to be surgically removed, while the effects of Depo-Provera may last for months. Thus these new technologies gave rise to the image of women on welfare kept sterile against their will.

Both birth-control methods also carry a high risk of side effects. Norplant-related suits have numbered in the hundreds, involving more than 50,000 women nationally. Depo-Provera was first developed in the 1970s, but it was banned in the United States then—even as U.S.- and UN-funded programs experimented with its use in Thailand, India, Colombia, Mexico, and Kenya. Some women, both in the United States and abroad, have complained that doctors will not remove Norplant even when asked repeatedly.

The controversy continued into the year 2000, when a controversial Michigan plan was revealed: Women with drug addictions were being offered $200 apiece to be sterilized. Once again, welfare rights activists and some feminist groups have charged that this is a particularly unfair way of targeting poor women and women of color.

In 2001, men, too, became the subjects of controversy involving reproductive rights and financial responsibility when the Wisconsin Supreme Court upheld a probation order barring a man convicted for failing to pay child support from having more children unless he showed that he could support all of his offspring. Wisconsin resident David Oaks, father of nine children by four women, owed $25,000 in child support. As a result of the ruling, Oaks faced up to eight years in prison if he violated the order. Even as policymakers concerned with "deadbeat dads" applauded the ruling, reproductive rights activists looked on with alarm, seeing the Wisconsin decision as heralding new levels of government intervention in people's reproductive freedom.

Genes, Clones, and Legal Tangles

The 1990s saw an explosion in genetic research and technology, from the Human Genome Project, a $3 billion undertaking funded by Congress in 1990 to map all the genes in the human cell; to the 1997 cloning of Dolly, the sheep. The decade abounded with colorful, improbable—and to some, horrifying—stories that seemed to be the stuff of either science fiction or TV courtroom drama: A 42-year-old woman carries a child for her daughter, giving birth to her own grandchild; fertility doctors secretly take eggs and embryos from childless women and use them to create children for other couples; a woman gives birth to twins of two different races because someone got the sperm mixed up during fertilization; a divorced couple fight over who gets custody of the frozen embryos they created when they were still married.

Despite the legal and medical tangles, fertility treatments continued to multiply. In 1997, U.S. doctors were writing 1.3 million fertility drug prescriptions per year, at a total cost of almost $230 million. In the same year, the first U.S. woman gave birth to a baby conceived from a frozen egg. Also in that year, an article in the prestigious scientific journal *Fertility and Sterility* reported on a South Korean study suggesting that freezing and thawing eggs may create chromosomal abnormalities in the children that result. Science reporters were torn between three kinds of stories: optimistic reports on new fertility treatments and discoveries; legal difficulties resulting from the new technology; and warnings from scientists, religious leaders, newspaper columnists, and others that new kinds of medical, social, and legal problems might lie ahead.

2000–2001 AND BEYOND

Stenberg v. Carhart and "Partial-Birth Abortion"

One of the major Supreme Court decisions came down in 2000: *Stenberg v. Carhart*, concerning a Nebraska bill outlawing so-called "partial-birth abortion." The court struck down the Nebraska law on the grounds that it violated *Roe v. Wade*, but the vote was only 5–4, and the four dissenters—Rehnquist, Thomas, Scalia, and White—explicitly said that they opposed *Roe* and would overturn it if they could. (Rehnquist and White had voted against *Roe* in the first place.) Pro-choice activists saw the vote as a sign of how close the Court was to abandoning *Roe*, so that even one pro-life nominee could turn the tide. When George W. Bush was elected a few months later, it seemed highly likely that the Court would soon turn against *Roe*.

The notion of "partial-birth abortion" was misleading in the first place—and part of why the Court overturned the Nebraska law. Supposedly, the law referred to a type of abortion procedure known as D&X—dilation and extraction—an extremely rare operation performed only in late-term abortions. However, the term "partial-birth" is not a medical term and might be construed to apply to procedures known as D&E—dilation and evacuation. In neither case is a child "born," although part of the fetus may emerge from the woman's body before the fetus is terminated.

Even supporters of the Nebraska law admitted that outlawing this method of abortion would not prevent abortion generally—only this particular procedure. In fact, according to the Centers for Disease Control, 88% of all abortions are performed during the first 12 weeks, and 91% during the first trimester, with only about 9% of all abortions performed during the second trimester. So D&X abortions were already a subset of a very small percentage of abortions. Data on D&X abortions are hotly contested, but estimates range from 0.02% of all abortions (only 450 per year) to almost 2%.

Most abortions performed in the second trimester, particularly later in the trimester, are the result of problems with either the pregnancy or the fetus, cases in which the woman believes that her life or health is at risk, or that the child she is carrying cannot survive normally. Pro-choice activists were enraged about what they saw as the hypocrisy of the Nebraska law. First, they argued, pro-life groups lobbied for waiting periods and closed clinics, so that women could not have safer and less traumatic early abortions. Then they wanted to penalize women who were forced to have later-term abortions.

Pro-life groups, on the other hand, described the D&X procedure in graphic terms that made it sound one step removed from infanticide. They argued that such a barbaric procedure should not be allowed; indeed, that it was beyond debate. (For more on this argument, see chapter 2.) It seemed that after *Stenberg v. Carhart*, however, pro-life groups were likely to turn their attention away from D&X abortions and to RU-486.

The "Abortion Pill"

On September 28, 2000, the FDA finally approved RU-486 (mifepristone), the "abortion pill," a hormonal medication that induces abortion in women who are within the first seven weeks of pregnancy. Although RU-486 had been legal in Europe for years, the FDA had delayed its approval in the United States—a move that pro-choice activists charged was a way of placating the pro-life movement. Pro-life activists, on the other hand, argued that the "abortion pill" was medically far more dangerous than supporters acknowledged and successfully lobbied for restrictions on the kinds of doctors who could prescribe it. Doctors not qualified to treat potential side effects are not allowed to write prescriptions for Mifeprex (the trade name of mifepristone, or RU-486), leading pro-choice columnist Katha Pollitt to wonder why similar restrictions are not in place for doctors prescribing Viagra, whose potential side effects include cardiac problems. Yet, Pollitt pointed out, no one had suggested that only heart specialists be allowed to prescribe the "potency pill" for men.

Pro-life activists have recently vowed to lobby for the same kinds of restrictions on RU-486 that they have successful imposed on abortion procedures: mandatory waiting periods, informed consent laws, restrictions to minors, and so on. According to NARAL, 257 anti-choice measures were introduced in 2000, of which 43 were enacted. Some 262 anti-choice measures have been enacted since 1995. So the possibility of anti-choice legislation against RU-486 would seem quite high, especially under a pro-life president. Abortion rights activists argue that RU-486 will be a special target of pro-life protestors, because taking RU-486 is so much more private than going to a clinic; thus, women's access to the pill will undermine clinic protest and other public pro-life activity.

The George W. Bush Administration

There was a great deal of confusion during the 2000 presidential campaign about George W. Bush's stand on abortion: People on both sides called him a moderate, while people on both sides also insisted that he was solidly pro-life. Although Bush has taken an ostensibly moderate line in his own rhetoric, his appointments have been passionately pro-life and generally conservative about the use of contraception. Bush's choice for attorney general was Missouri senator John Ashcroft, while his pick as secretary of Health and Human Services was Wisconsin governor Tommy Thompson. Both are well-known as outspoken opponents of abortion, although during his confirmation hearings, Ashcroft pledged to support *Roe v. Wade* as long as it was the settled law of the land.

Bush also chose Wade Horn to head the welfare agency within Thompson's department, drawing fire from many women's, welfare rights, and reproductive rights groups. Horn was a controversial figure for his 1997 support of a plan to give married couples preferential treatments for such public benefits as housing and Head Start (a program for preschool children at risk of doing poorly in school), a plan that women's groups criticized for tending to trap poor women into abusive marriages, as well as being unconstitutional. Horn renounced these views in his Senate confirmation hearings, but he continued to preach abstinence-only sex education and suggested offering young women at risk of getting pregnant a $5,000 bonus for deferring childbirth until after marriage.

Bush also nominated E. Anne Peterson to head global programs at the U.S. Agency for International Development (USAID). Peterson, a former health commissioner in the state of Virginia, was well known for her opposition to widening the availability of emergency contraception, the so-called morning-after pill. Such contraception is often used by women in refugee camps, where rapes and sexual assaults happen frequently. As of fall 2001, Bush was considering the nomination of John Klink to head the State Department's Bureau of Population, Refugees, and Migration. Klink, a devout Roman Catholic currently employed as a diplomat with the Vatican mission to the United Nations (UN), has drawn fire for his strong convictions against abortion, emergency contraception, and the use of condoms to halt the spread of AIDS. Pro-choice and women's groups strongly opposed his nomination, while conservative and Catholic organiztions supported it. Pro-choice Secretary of State Colin Powell also reportedly expressed his outrage at the possiblity of Klink's nomination.

Bush's foreign policy has been marked by a strong opposton to abortion and contraception from his first day in office. Virtually his first official act as president was to ban federal aid to international organizations that perform or "actively promote" abortion as a family planning method. He reinstituted a gag rule that President Clinton had lifted: No clinic that even mentions abortion as a possibility—even in countries where abortion is legal—can receive U.S. funds. Congress sought to find a way around Bush's action, even as the pro-choice Center for Reproductive Law and Policy brought suit in Manhattan Federal District Court, arguing that the rights of free speech and political association were violated by the president's order. President Bush, meanwhile, continued to look for other legal means of imposing abortion restrictions on foreign aid, in an effort to prevent Congress from overturning his action of January 22. He also moved to reverse President Clinton's UN policies, inviting pro-life groups that had formerly been shut out of UN and World Health Organization (WHO) meetings to serve as part of official U.S. delegations.

Domestically, Bush also made some moves that some believed were a harbinger of future actions to curtail abortion rights. In July, the draft of a letter by Dennis Smith, director of the Center for Medicaid and State Operations, was leaked to the press, suggesting that fetuses would be defined as "unborn children" so that low-income women who did not qualify for Medicaid would be able to receive federal coverage for insurance. Reproductive rights groups were outraged by the move, which they saw as a "back door" move to create legal rights for fetuses, including their own right to health care, while pro-life groups supported the idea.

48

Bush's election came in the wake of intensified national debate about abortion. On October 21, 1999, the Senate voted 51–47 to affirm *Roe v. Wade*. Yet one month earlier, on September 30, 1999, the House of Representatives voted 254–172 to support HR 2436, the so-called Unborn Victims of Violence Act, a bill that would grant fetuses legal standing with rights separate and equal to that of the women carrying them. The House law was part of a trend towards "fetal rights": seeing the fetus as a legal and moral person with rights equal to the pregnant woman. In April 1999, for example, a Louisiana Senate judiciary committee had passed a law giving an embryo the right to sue from the point of conception on. These developments were momentous enough under a pro-choice president, who would likely have vetoed any federal legislation calling for "fetal rights." What will a pro-life president do with a congressional fetal rights bill?

When Bush went into office, pro-choice sentiment was at its lowest point in several years. According to a *Los Angeles Times* poll conducted in June 2000, only 43% of the people surveyed said they supported *Roe v. Wade*, down from 56% in 1991. Some 65% of the respondents and 72% of the female respondents, said that abortion should not be available in the second trimester. A full 46% said that abortion should be legal only in cases of rape, incest, and to save the mother's life; and 8% said it should be always illegal. How this national sentiment will affect a Bush presidency remains to be seen.

However, one indication of Congress's possible role in the debate came in October 2001, when Louisiana Republican representative David Vitter proposed an amendment to a spending bill that would deny federal family-planning funds to groups that perform abortions. Vitter's amendment would in effect extend President Bush's ruling on family planning funds abroad to clinics and other organizations at home. Title X of the Public Health Act provides $250 million in family planning funds each year, about 40% of which goes to private agencies. Since about half of these groups perform abortions, they would no longer receive federal funds if Vitter's amendment were passed. NARAL has expressed dismay over the proposed amendment, estimating that some 1 million women would lose their family planning services under the Vitter plan. While the future of Vitter's plan is uncertain, it suggests that further such actions may be a feature of Congressional activities in the coming years.

Hospital Mergers

Another factor that will likely influence reproductive rights is the trend toward hospital mergers. A July 2000 *Redbook* article pointed out that between 1995 and 2000, 132 nonsectarian hospitals had merged with Catholic institutions and would therefore no longer perform abortions, tubal ligations, and fertility procedures, all of which Catholic teachings oppose. The *Redbook* article profiled Kathleen Hutchins, who felt her water break in the fourteenth week of pregnancy and was told by her ob/gyn that she was unlikely to be able to carry her baby to term. Even if she did, the doctor said—which would require six months of bed rest and a highly uncertain outcome—there was only a 2% chance that the baby would survive. Moreover, if the fetus died inside Hutchins, it might cause an effect that could require a hysterectomy or even cause Hutchins's death. Her doctor advised her to complete the miscarriage that had begun naturally by having an emergency abortion and expelling the fetus.

However, the hospital where her doctor usually sent his patients had recently merged with the only other hospital in Hutchins's hometown of Manchester, New Hampshire—Catholic Medical Center. The doctor arranged for an abortion at another hospital—but the nearest facility was 80 miles away, and Hutchins had no way to get there. When the doctor tried to defy the hospital administration, he was threatened with a loss of hospital privileges and told that anyone who assisted him would be fired. In the end, his practice paid $400 for a taxi to take his patient to the other hospital.

The *Redbook* article went on to cite a study by Catholics for a Free Choice, who had reviewed 36 of the 43 Catholic-secular mergers completed in 1998. Almost half of these joint health centers had responded to the mergers by eliminating some or all of the reproductive services formerly offered. The Catholic Health Association of the United States called the study "misleading," but says that it has no comparable analysis. Pro-choice activists are so concerned about the trend that they have started a watchdog group, MergerWatch. In many communities, mergers are now being opposed by coalitions of local groups.

Birth Control Coverage

Another major reproductive rights issue that arose in 2001 was the question of insurance coverage for contraception. Since 1998, some 13 states enacted prescription equity laws, requiring that insurance companies pay for birth control if they paid for other similar things. These laws have been a source of controversy: Many states are considering passing similar laws, even as birth control coverage has been the subject of several lawsuits. In June, for example, a Seattle federal judge ruled that a family-owned drugstore chain discriminated against women when it failed to include prescription contraceptions in its employee health plan. The Seattle case was the result of a class-action lawsuit filed in July 2000 by Jennifer Erickson, a pharmacist at Bartell Drug Company. Erickson claimed that the company's health insurance plan violated the Pregnancy Discrimination Act, because the plan provided for all the health needs of male employees, even as female employees had to pay for their own contraception. Then, in July, a California state appeals court upheld a state law requiring employers to cover contraceptives in their prescription drug plans. The law had been challenged by Catholic Charities, who had argued that the law infringed on the religious freedom of employers. Inspired by these actions, the Washington state chapter of NARAL and the American Civil Liberties Union (ACLU) also brought suit against the Seattle-based Regence BlueShield insurance company, in an effort to require it to cover prescription contraceptives. It seems likely that the controversy will continue in many other states.

Infertility Treatments: Many Questions Remain

As reproductive technology moves into the twenty-first century, feminists, scientists, and other observers continue to raise questions about infertility: How big is the problem, what causes it, what can—or should—be done about it. The Centers for Disease Control and Prevention have estimated that infertility affects 6.1 million couples, or 10% to 15% of people of reproductive age. In other words, about 1 in every 10 couples is infertile—and this figure is expected to rise as ever more women postpone childbearing to pursue their careers. Infertility has been portrayed as a pressing problem, leading many women—and men—to become desperate for new treatments that will enable them to conceive and/or bear children. But Janice Raymond, author of *Women as Wombs*, argues that part of women's desperation is caused by social pressures that view being childless as abnormal. She quotes a letter writer to *Ms.* magazine who "concludes that there would be fewer ethical dilemmas created by the use of reproductive technologies if people accepted infertility and did not pressure the infertile to have a child at any cost."

Both Raymond and reproductive technology expert Lori Andrews have also argued that success figures for fertility treatments are vastly exaggerated. In some cases, they argue, clinics find ways of misrepresenting their success; for example, they tell new patients about the ratio between the numbers of babies they've helped create and their total number of patients, without revealing that many of the babies born were twins or triplets.

Moreover, the optimistic tone of most science reporting suggests that IVF and other treatments have a near-100% success rate, instead of the far lower figures that are actually true. The latest figures available are from a 1998 Centers for Disease Control (CDC) study: 360 fertility clinics helped produce more than 28,000 babies conceived in 1998 (and born in 1998 and 1999). According to the CDC, IVF was up 12%, to 77,013 attempts in 1998 from 68,615 in 1997. Women under 35 seeking to get pregnant with their own eggs saw success rates rise from 35.9% in 1997 to 37.3% in 1998; success rates overall were approximately 25%. Another report suggests that for women over 40, the success rate is closer to 10%. No data is available on the average number of cycles that an individual woman goes through to achieve success, though doctors agree that for most women, it takes more than one try, with each cycle costing from $8,000 to $12,000.

Other problems raised by Andrews, Raymond, and science writer Ann Pappert include the health risks caused by multiple births, the extent to which new treatments are tried out on women without sufficient testing, and the lack of long-term data on children who were created by these new means. Pappert has also speculated about the risks of ovarian cancer from ovulation-induction treatments.

New Legal Battles

In the summer of 2001, a number of new legal issues arose concerning both fertility medicine and the consequences of assisted conception and birth. In July, for example, the FDA announced that a controversial type of fertility treatment would now come under its regulation. While the FDA had always maintained that it had the power to regulate fertility treatments, this was the first time it had chosen to exercise that power. The regulations concerned a technique in which fluids from a young, fertile woman's egg are injected into the egg of an older, infertile woman's egg before the older woman's egg is fertilized by her partner's sperm, leading to the unprecedented mixing of three kinds of genetic material rather than two. The procdeure was pioneered by Barnabas Medical Center in Livingston, New Jersey, but some half-dozen clinics offer the procedure, a number that will probably grow as the method gains acceptance.

In August, the New Jersey Supreme Court upheld a woman's right to decide whether frozen embryos produced by her and her ex-husband through IVF during their marriage could be implanted into another woman. The court ruled that the seven embryos produced by the couple could not be used to create a child without the woman's consent. Anti-abortion groups, which had long maintained that embryos represent life, were disappointed in the ruling, while reproductive rights groups supported the ruling.

Then, in September, the Massachusetts hight court, the Supreme Judicial Court, heard a case about whether children conceived posthumously from their late father's frozen sperm were eligible for Social Security benefits. The Social Security Administration had ruled that because the twins were born after the father's death, an 1836 state law required them to be considered illegitimate. Also in September, the U.S. 9th Circuit Court of Appeals ruled that male prisoners have a constitutional right to procreate by means of artificial insemination. The suit had been brought by William Reno Gerber, a 41-year-old third-time convict serving an 111-year sentence for negligently discharging a firearm, making terrorist threats, and possessing a handgun as an ex-felon. Gerber wanted to send a semen sample to a medical center in Chicago, to be used to impregnate his 46-year-old wife. The ruling was supported by civil liberties groups, who cited a 1978 Supreme Court ruling allowing prisoners to marry. It was opposed by some conservatives, who raised eugenic arguments, among them Sacramento lawyer Ron Zumbrun, founder of the Pacific Legal Foundation, who asked, "If you are having lifetime criminals furthering their genes, is that in the best interests of society?" And in Massachusetts, the Supreme Judicial Court heard the case of Marla and Steven Culliton, the genetic parents of twins that were carried during pregnancy and borne by a surrogate who had no interest in raising them. Despite the surrogate's wish that Cullitons act as the parents of their genetic child, the Cullitons were not given the parental rights they sought before their children were born, with the probate judge ruling that adoption law prevents birth mothers from legally giving up their parental rights before birth.

The Culliton case offered the possibility that surrogacy law might come to be better defined as the number of surrogate births increases. Currently, 26 states have laws governing surrogacy, with at least four states—Michigan, New York, Utah, and Washington—banning it outright; others have simply regulated it in various ways.

Ethical and Legal Questions

As fertility treatments become more commonplace, a number of ethical, legal, and social questions have arisen. While a full discussion of these concerns is beyond the scope of this book, here is an overview of the kinds of questions that remain—and that loom ever larger for the future:

- *Custody issues.* How should custody be determined when multiple parents are involved? For example, who should get custody of a child with two adoptive parents, an egg donor, a sperm donor, and a surrogate mother? What happens when contracts are made between parents and surrogates or donors under certain circumstances—and then those circumstances change? What if the adoptive parents get divorced, or the child born has mental or physical problems? Should the contract still hold? What about the custody of frozen embryos?

- *Financial issues.* Currently only 12 states mandate insurance coverage for infertility treatments, but advocates seek to raise this number. Should fertility be considered a medical "right" for which others should pay?

- *Genetic manipulation.* Is there a difference between screening prospective children for genetic diseases and screening them for eye color or height—or gender? Is it ethical to create a child specifically in order to be a blood donor or a bone-marrow donor for another child?

- *Scientific research.* Is science being driven by the marketplace, with millions of dollars going for high-tech fertility treatments and little going for low-cost effective birth control? Is science being driven by social ideas, so that most fertility treatments and birth control involve women, not men? Is science being driven by politics, so that stem-cell research on embryos is off-limits because of right-to-life activism? Is it good for science to be affected by these other factors? Should science be regulated more, less, or not at all?

- *Egg and sperm donation.* Should donors be paid, and if so, how much? Should donations be regulated, or should society accept phenomena like the $24.95/month web site set up by a former *Playboy* photographer offering the eggs of beautiful women at higher prices? Should women be able to get information on the identity of sperm donors? Should such information be available to children created by the sperm? Should donors be able to locate the children they helped create? If a sperm donor has a medical condition that causes problems for the child, should he be liable for a suit? Should the sperm bank? How does it affect children to grow up knowing that they were created through egg and/or sperm donation? Should donors, surrogates, and children be able to have ongoing relationships, or should the child be acquainted only with the adoptive parent(s)?

- *Family life and gender roles.* Once families are no longer tied to genetic reproduction, does that change the nature of the family? Does it alter women's roles? Men's roles? Is there something valuable about the traditional family that society should seek to identify and preserve? Is there something valuable about the newly possible "multiple" families that society should seek to identify and foster?

- *International issues.* What's the relationship between ever more advanced fertility treatments in the United States and lack of funds for family planning in many other parts of the world? To what extent are fertility and other medications tested on women in developing nations and/or U.S. women on welfare before they are approved for all U.S. women? What are the implications of the growing global market for eggs and sperm, which are currently being traded worldwide at enormous profit, according to articles in both the *Wall Street Journal* and the *Christian Science Monitor?*

None of these questions have easy answers; maybe some of these questions have no answers at all. But as the coming decade proceeds, one thing is certain: society will face these troubling questions. One way or another, the questions raised by reproductive rights and technology will continue to affect the lives of many.

CHAPTER 2

THE LAW OF REPRODUCTIVE RIGHTS AND TECHNOLOGY

THE LAW OF REPRODUCTIVE TECHNOLOGY

Although reproductive technology has been posing troubling legal questions for some years now, the law of reproductive technology is still very much in its infancy. Indeed, legal scholars such as Lori B. Andrews have expressed their alarm that reproductive issues remain largely unregulated by either the state or the federal government.

The major arena in which reproductive law has been forged by the courts is in the form of civil suits brought by various parents or would-be parents objecting to their treatment by doctors and fertility clinics or seeking custody of children created by new reproductive means.

Yet although there have been many well-known cases—which often are later portrayed in fictional form on TV courtroom dramas—few legal principles have emerged from this courtroom activity. Whether a surrogate has the right to keep a newborn child despite the existence of a contract requiring her to give it up; whether a man has the right to insist that his wife destroy embryos that the two of them created together; whether a woman can insist on child support from a man who donated sperm to another woman who intends to give the child to the first woman after birth—all of these are questions that have been the subjects of suits, and yet have not established any firm national precedent for how to resolve these matters.

Therefore, information about key suits involving reproductive technology may be found in chapter 3, the Chronology, while the bulk of this chapter will be devoted to the law of reproductive rights.

THE LAW OF REPRODUCTIVE RIGHTS

An enormous amount of legal action has been taken on reproductive rights: dozens of Supreme Court decisions, numerous national and state laws, and a variety of regulations that all affect the extent to which various women have access to contraception and abortion. Moreover, the legal situation is constantly changing, as new laws are written and new court cases are brought.

This chapter, therefore, concentrates on two major aspects of reproductive rights law: the four major Supreme Court decisions on abortion and a state-by-state summary of reproductive rights. Every modern Supreme Court decision on abortion and contraception is described briefly in chapter 3, the Chronology. Here, the four major decisions on abortion are analyzed, including both majority and minority opinions so that readers can follow the thinking about abortion that has shaped the national legal climate.

But reproductive rights is far more than a matter of what the Supreme Court says. The situation in each state is different, and different kinds of women—especially low-income women and minors—are affected differently. Therefore, the Supreme Court Cases section is followed by a Summary of State Laws and Regulations Regarding Abortion and Contraception, which explains exactly what kinds of restrictions on abortion and contraception were in force in late 2001 in each of the 50 states.

SUPREME COURT CASES

ROE V. WADE (1973)

Background

At issue in *Roe v. Wade* was a Texas statute criminalizing abortion: Texas Penal Code, Article 1196. Texas first made abortion illegal in 1854. Although modifications were made to the statute in 1857, 1866, 1879, and 1911, the law remained basically the same: Abortion was illegal except when there had been "medical advice for the purpose of saving the life of the mother."

In March 1970, a young, single, pregnant woman named Norma McCorvey decided to challenge that law. Under the pseudonym of Jane Roe (significantly, McCorvey took a false name to protect herself against the stigma of being an unwed mother), she brought suit against Henry Wade, the district attorney in Dallas County, where she lived. McCorvey/Roe sought a declaratory judgment—a conclusive, binding statement by the court—that the Texas criminal abortion statutes were unconstitutional. She also wanted an injunction preventing the D.A. from enforcing the anti-abortion statute.

56

In her suit, McCorvey/Roe said that she wanted to end her pregnancy via an abortion "performed by a competent, licensed physician, under safe, clinical conditions." She readily acknowledged that her life was not threatened by her pregnancy, but she did not want to bear a child, and she could not afford to travel to a place where abortion was legal.

McCorvey was already pregnant when she brought her suit to federal district court in March 1970, and she realized that by the time the case was over, her own access to abortion would probably be moot. However, she had her attorney, Sarah Weddington, add an amendment to her complaint, explaining that she was suing "on behalf of herself and all other women" in the same situation.

Legal Issues

McCorvey argued that the Texas laws on abortion were unconstitutionally vague—that is, they were written in such a way that they could not be applied fairly, since "medical advice" was such an unspecific term. For more than a century, every U.S. state had criminalized abortion but had allowed exceptions if a doctor found that the woman's life would be endangered by the pregnancy. Some doctors interpreted this to mean that the woman's life had to be in physical danger; others took a more lenient view, finding that a pregnancy might endanger a woman's mental health or interfere with the quality of her life. Because the Texas law was so vague, a woman's access to abortion might simply depend on whether she could find the right doctor.

McCorvey/Roe also argued that the Texas statute interfered with her right of personal privacy—her right to make her own medical decisions—which she claimed was protected by the First, Fourth, Fifth, Ninth, and Fourteenth Amendments. (The First Amendment guarantees freedom of speech and religion. The Fourth protects against unreasonable search and seizure of property. The Fifth holds that a person cannot be compelled to testify against her- or himself. The Ninth Amendment points out that people might have rights that go beyond those explicitly specified in the Constitution. And the Fourteenth Amendment guarantees that every citizen is entitled to an equal opportunity to "due process" under the law. That is, every citizen must have the equal protection of the law; no citizen or group of citizens can be treated by the law as a special case.)

In the words of the majority opinion that Justice Harry Blackmun wrote for the Court, Roe was arguing that the Texas statutes "improperly invade[d] . . . the concept of personal 'liberty' embodied in the Fourteenth Amendment's Due Process Clause . . . [and the] personal, marital, familial, and sexual privacy said to be protected by the Bill of Rights. . . ."

Decision

The first issue that the Court had to address was whether Roe even had the right to bring suit. In his opinion for the Court, Blackmun pointed out that since Roe's 1970 pregnancy had certainly ended by the time of his decision in 1973, the case was in one sense moot. However, he said, most pregnancies would be over by the time the cases involving them had been heard. If courts insisted upon hearing pregnancy-related cases only when the plaintiff was actually pregnant, there would never be any rulings on pregnancy-related issues. Besides, he wrote, even though Roe was no longer pregnant, the issues she raised would affect other women, and might affect her, too, if she became pregnant again. Therefore, the Court was going to hear Roe's case.

Blackmun then went on to review the history of U.S. laws about abortion and the place of abortion in Western civilization generally. He wrote that abortion was not barred by "ancient religion," such as that practiced by the Egyptians, Greeks, and Romans. Although the Hippocratic Oath forbade abortion, it represented only a small segment of ancient Greek opinion, according to Blackmun. Common law—the unwritten law followed in England, which is the basis for much U.S. jurisprudence—allowed abortion to be performed before quickening: "the first recognizable movement of the fetus in utero, appearing usually from the 16th to the 18th week of pregnancy." And perhaps, Blackmun pointed out, abortion might not be considered a crime under common law even after the fetus had quickened.

Blackmun went on to quote modern English law, which was generally liberal with regard to abortion, and U.S. law, which until the mid-nineteenth century had followed English common law in allowing early abortions. Thus, Blackmun wrote, "[T]hroughout the major portion of the 19th century, . . . a woman enjoyed a substantially broader right to terminate a pregnancy than she does in most States [sic] today."

Blackmun then reviewed the positions of the American Medical Association (AMA), the American Public Health Association (APHA), and the American Bar Association (ABA). He discussed the historical reasons why abortion had been criminalized in the nineteenth century, pointing out that there were no longer any important *medical* reasons to ban abortion, as the procedure had become much safer.

The fact that Blackmun went so thoroughly into the historical and social background of abortion is significant. It showed that he and the Court realized that they were ruling on an issue far greater than one of legal interpretation. The question at hand was not simply what the Constitution did or did not allow. It was whether the Supreme Court was willing to rule in a way that legalized nationwide access to abortion. To justify the ruling, Blackmun seemed to find it necessary to discuss abortion in the broadest possible context, showing that many societies and respectable organizations did not view it as criminal.

Finally, Blackmun proceeded to the actual legal issue: the question of privacy, which Roe had claimed as the centerpiece of her argument. He wrote:

> *The Constitution does not explicitly mention any right of privacy. . . . [However,] the Court has recognized that a right of personal privacy, or a guarantee of certain areas or zones of privacy, does exist under the Constitution. . . . This right of privacy . . . is broad enough to encompass a woman's decision whether or not to terminate her pregnancy. . . . We, therefore, conclude that the right of personal privacy includes the abortion decision . . .*

Blackmun and the Court majority found that women's right to privacy did indeed include the right to have an abortion. But the decision included some important restrictions on abortion rights as well. Roe had argued "that the woman's right is absolute and that she is entitled to terminate her pregnancy at whatever time, in whatever way, and for whatever reason she alone chooses." But, wrote Blackmun, "With this we do not agree. . . . The Court's decisions recognizing a right of privacy also acknowledge that some state regulation in areas protected by that right is appropriate."

What kind of state regulation might be appropriate? Blackmun wrote that the State had a "compelling reason" to safeguard health, maintain medical standards, and to protect potential life. True, in this particular case, the district attorney had not shown that the Texas law was justified by any of these considerations. But that did not mean that anti-abortion laws could never be justified—just that the Texas law could not be justified.

Blackmun went on to review both D.A. Wade's opinion and Roe's. Wade, he pointed out, had argued that the fetus is a "person," so that fetuses also deserved equal protection under the law. Blackmun found this unpersuasive. Although the Constitution did not actually define personhood, his reading of it suggested that "the word 'person,' as used in the Fourteenth Amendment, does not include the unborn."

On the other hand, Blackmun wrote,

> *The pregnant woman cannot be isolated in her privacy. She carries an embryo and later, a fetus. . . . As we have intimated above, it is reasonable and appropriate for a State to decide that at some point in time another interest, that of the health of the mother or that of potential human life, becomes significantly involved. The woman's privacy is no longer sole and any right of privacy she possesses must be measured accordingly.*

In other words, both a woman's health and the potential life of a fetus were legitimate concerns of the state.

With regard to a woman's health, Blackmun wrote, the State's interest in protecting the health of the mother began at the end of the first trimester. He picked this point on the grounds that a first-trimester abortion was safer, medically, than childbirth. Therefore, after the first trimester,

> . . . *a State may regulate the abortion procedure to the extent that the regulation reasonably relates to the preservation and protection of maternal health.*

For example, Blackmun wrote, a state could set requirements for the qualifications of the person performing the abortion; that person's licensing; the facility where the procedure would be performed (hospital, clinic, or somewhere else); the facility's licensing, and so on.

Thus, Blackmun explained, during the first trimester, a doctor and patient could determine, free from State regulation, whether an abortion should be conducted. After the first trimester, in the patient's interest, the State could regulate abortion procedures.

What about the State's compelling interest in protecting "potential life"? Texas law had answered this question by finding that life began at conception and was present throughout pregnancy. But Blackmun explicitly refused to consider the question of when life began. "When those trained in . . . medicine, philosophy, and theology are unable to arrive at any consensus, the judiciary . . . is not in a position to speculate as to the answer."

Instead, Blackmun wrote, he would simply rule that the State's interest in fetal life—and thus its ability to regulate abortions—began at the point of "viability," the point at which the fetus could survive outside the womb. He explicitly stated that the government could outlaw abortion as soon as the fetus was viable:

> *If the State is interested in protecting fetal life after viability, it may go so far as to proscribe [prohibit] abortion during that period, except when it is necessary to preserve the life or health of the mother.*

However, the Texas law did not limit itself to protecting women after the first trimester and fetuses after viability. Instead, it simply outlawed abortion altogether, except when a doctor said that the pregnant woman's life was in danger. Blackmun found that the Texas statute was far too sweeping, and therefore, he overturned it.

Chief Justice Warren Burger wrote a concurring (agreeing) opinion, although he found himself "somewhat troubled that the Court has taken notice of various scientific and medical data in reaching its conclusion." Burger would have preferred for the decision to have been reached on purely legal grounds.

Like Blackmun, Burger felt that "States must have broad power, within the limits indicated in the opinions, to regulate the subject of abortion"; also like Burger, he felt that the Texas regulations were too sweeping. He personally would have liked the State "to require the certification of two physicians to support an abortion," but, he added ruefully, "the Court holds otherwise."

Justice William O. Douglas likewise agreed with the opinion, and likewise noted that "The protection of the fetus when it has acquired life is a legitimate concern of the State." Justice Potter Stewart, also agreeing, wrote that the State had the right not only to regulate abortions, but "to regulate abortions more stringently [than other surgical procedures] or even to prohibit them in the late stages of pregnancy." Nevertheless, like the rest of the majority, he found the Texas law too broad to be constitutional. Justices Thurgood Marshall and Lewis Powell voted with the majority without writing their own opinions.

Dissenting were Justices Byron White and William Rehnquist. White wrote the minority opinion. When he summarized the majority opinion, he wrote disparagingly:

> [The majority finds that] the Constitution of the United States values the convenience, whim, or caprice of the putative mother more than the life or potential life of the fetus . . . With all due respect, I dissent . . . The Court simply fashions and announces a new constitutional right for pregnant mothers and, with scarcely any reason or authority for its action, invests that right with sufficient substance to override most existing state abortion statutes. . . . The Court apparently values the convenience of the pregnant mother more than the continued existence and development of the life or potential life that she carries . . .

In other words, White argued, the Court had exceeded its authority. Rather than sticking strictly to the Constitution, it had found within the Constitution a right for pregnant women that simply was not there—and then had used that spurious "right" to assert that state abortion statutes were not valid.

However he personally felt about whose rights took precedence—the woman's or the fetus's—White wrote, he could find "no constitutional warrant" for imposing a particular opinion on the U.S. people, no evidence that the Constitution required states to value the woman's "whim" over the fetus's "potential life." Instead of the Supreme Court stepping in and claiming constitutional authority, White argued, "this issue . . . should be left with the people" and the governments they elected.

Reproductive Rights and Technology

Rehnquist found it inappropriate that the Court had written a decision based on the complaint of a pregnant woman who, for all they knew, might have been in her last trimester of pregnancy when she filed her complaint. Since by the majority's own opinion, Texas had the right to outlaw abortions in the last trimester, perhaps the Texas law was appropriate where Roe was concerned.

What if Roe had been in her first trimester when she brought suit? Even then, Rehnquist argued, the most the Court should have done was rule that the anti-abortion law had been inappropriately applied to her. The Texas law itself was not unconstitutional, in Rehnquist's view; only—perhaps—its application to Roe. Therefore, Rehnquist said, the Court should not have used Roe's suit "as a fulcrum" for making broader decisions about abortion.

Nor did Rehnquist agree that Roe's right of privacy was at issue. He was not persuaded by her argument that abortion was a fundamental right. On the contrary, Rehnquist wrote, most states had restricted abortions for at least 100 years. That was the true measure of where the American people stood on this issue. Therefore, he argued,

> . . . the asserted right to an abortion is not "so rooted in the traditions and conscience of our people as to be ranked as fundamental." Even today, when society's views on abortion are changing, the very existence of the debate is evidence that the "right" to an abortion is not so universally accepted as [Roe] would have us believe.

Moreover, Rehnquist argued with some asperity, the Supreme Court's decision in *Roe v. Wade* was ultimately unclear and provided insufficient guidance for lawmakers. He wrote, ". . . [T]he Court's opinion will accomplish the seemingly impossible feat of leaving this area of the law more confused than it found it."

Impact

Between 1973, when *Roe* was decided, and 1979, only six years later, the number of legal abortions performed on U.S. women aged 15–44 nearly doubled, from 744,600 in 1973 to 1,497,700 in 1979. The increase is even more dramatic for women in their twenties: from 370,200 abortions in 1973 to 809,900 in 1979. In the three decades since *Roe*, U.S. women have continued to have abortions at virtually the same annual rate, a major impact of the Court's decision to overturn the Texas statute and all others like it.

Moreover, *Roe* created a new climate both for those who supported a woman's right to have an abortion and for those who opposed it. Whereas antiabortion or "pro-life" activism occurred sporadically and on a local level before 1973, the *Roe* decision spawned a nationwide movement. (See chapter 1.) From political lobbying to the murder of abortion providers, from a national cultural campaign to the picketing of local clinics, from politicians' speeches to direct-mail campaigns, the right-to-life issue has been a central feature of U.S. politics ever since *Roe v. Wade*. Even Norma McCorvey, the young woman who brought the suit and called herself "Roe," became a right-to-life activist, claiming that the feminists who helped her sue the Dallas D.A. had used and manipulated her.

The language used by the Justices on both sides of *Roe* has continued to shape the abortion debate and has affected other questions of reproductive rights as well. Because even the majority Justices stressed the state's right to regulate late-term abortions, it has been easier for later legal decisions to encroach upon the "absolute" right to choose that Roe sought and that the Court denied. The fact that the majority opinion refused to consider the question of when life begins has made it far more difficult for this issue to be inserted into later legal language—although the notion of "fetal rights" has gained some ground in the 1990s and early twenty-first century. Both in what it allowed and in what it did not allow, the language of *Roe* set the boundaries for the debates that followed. (See chapter 1.)

Meanwhile, making early-term abortions legal meant that women no longer needed to turn to illegal providers, the so-called back-alley abortionists that had been such a central image in the "right to choose" campaigns. Nor did women need to abort themselves with such dangerous means as coat hangers and household bleach. Thus, another impact of *Roe* was that thousands of women's lives were saved, as women exercised their new right to safe and legal abortions.

At the same time, a woman's right not to bear a child had a profoundly transformative effect on women's and men's views of motherhood, femininity, and female sexuality. The notion that a woman's sexual activity could be viewed separately from her ability to procreate led to new ways of seeing women's roles in the workplace, at home, and in the bedroom. For many in the pro-life movement, these were disturbing developments. Others greeted the changes with enthusiasm. (See chapter 1.) In either case, new ways of understanding womanhood and motherhood flowed from the decision to allow women even the partial right to terminate their pregnancies.

WEBSTER V. REPRODUCTIVE HEALTH SERVICES (1989)

Background

Ever since the landmark decision of *Roe v. Wade* in 1973, opponents of abortion had looked for ways to limit women's access to abortion. On federal, state, and local levels, they had tried to ban the use of public funds to pay for abortions or for abortion-related counseling; instituted mandatory waiting periods and/or counseling before a woman could have an abortion; and regulated the circumstances under which an abortion could be performed (e.g., only in a hospital, only before a certain time in the pregnancy, etc.). Some of these efforts at restricting access to abortion survived court challenges, and some did not.

In June 1986, the governor of Missouri signed into law a bill known as Missouri Senate Committee Substitute for House Bill No. 1596, which amended existing state law regarding abortions and prenatal care. The act included 20 provisions, 4 of which were the subject of a Supreme Court hearing in 1989:

1. a preamble stating "findings" by the state legislature that "[t]he life of each human being begins at conception" and that "unborn children have protectable interests in life, health and well-being";
2. a requirement that before performing an abortion on any woman who might be at least 20 weeks pregnant, doctors should determine whether the fetus was viable by performing "such medical examinations and tests as are necessary to make a finding of the gestational age [how old the fetus was], weight, and lung maturity of the unborn child";
3. a prohibition against using public employees or facilities to perform abortions not needed to save the woman's life;
4. a prohibition against using public funds, employees, or facilities to "encourag[e] or counsel" a woman to have an abortion not needed to save her life.

In July 1986, three doctors, a nurse, a social worker, Planned Parenthood of Kansas City, and Reproductive Health Services brought a class action suit in U.S. District Court, claiming that the statute was not constitutional because some of its provisions violated the First, Fourth, Ninth, and Fourteenth Amendments. They argued that the statute violated the "privacy rights of pregnant women seeking abortions"; women's "right to an abortion"; the "righ[t] to privacy in the physician-patient relationship"; a doctor's right "to practice medicine"; pregnant women's "right to life due to inherent risks involved in childbirth"; and women's right to "receive . . . adequate medical advice and treatment" concerning abortions.

All of the individuals bringing suit worked at public health facilities in Missouri; all engaged in counseling that included explaining the option of abortion to women and helping them to make use of that option if they chose. Two of the three doctors in the suit actually performed abortions at public hospitals. Since public hospitals tended to be used by low-income women and women without health insurance, the plaintiffs felt that this law discriminated against poor women, making it harder for them to obtain the full range of services that a middle-class woman at a private hospital might get. They also felt that the legislature should not be restricting them from providing the kind of counseling and medical services that they thought their clients needed.

Planned Parenthood of Kansas City provided counseling and family planning for women, including abortions for women up to 14 weeks pregnant. Reproductive Health Services offered similar services, providing abortions up to 22 weeks into the pregnancy. Both were nonprofit corporations.

Legal Issues

Initially, the courts seemed to favor the plaintiffs. The District Court ruled that the law could not be enforced until after a trial, which was held in December 1986. At that time, the court found seven provisions of the act unconstitutional and ruled that they could not be enforced. These seven provisions included the four already described, plus a statement that unborn children had the same rights as other persons; a requirement that doctors inform pregnant women of certain facts before performing abortions; and a rule stating that abortions after week 16 of pregnancy could only be performed in hospitals. (Supporters of abortion rights objected to rules requiring that earlier-term abortions be performed in hospitals. They claimed that such provisions were not medically necessary; they only made abortions more expensive and harder to obtain.)

The District Court's rulings were affirmed by the Court of Appeals for the Eighth Circuit. But William Webster, Missouri's attorney general, decided to take the case all the way to the Supreme Court. By the time the Supreme Court ruled, only four sections of the Missouri law were involved: 1) the preamble; 2) the prohibition against the use of public facilities or employees to perform abortions; 3) the prohibition against the use of public funds for counseling that mentioned abortions as a possible option; 4) the requirement that doctors conduct tests of fetuses 20 weeks old or older, to determine whether they were viable.

At the time of the case, scientists generally agreed that the earliest possible time when a fetus might be viable was $23^1/_2$ to 24 weeks. However, defenders of the law pointed out that women did not always know exactly when they had gotten pregnant. So a woman who thought she was 20 weeks pregnant might be carrying an older—and viable—fetus. Since *Roe v. Wade* had found that the State might protect the lives of viable fetuses, it was permissible—even crucial—to determine whether any fetus to be aborted was in fact viable.

Critics of the act pointed out that requiring doctors to perform tests on all women pregnant for 20 weeks or more meant that unnecessary and expensive tests would add to the trouble and cost of an abortion; would force women to get abortions later in their pregnancies, when abortions were more dangerous and more traumatic; interfered with the wishes of individual patients and the judgment of individual doctors; and might endanger the life of the woman. They argued that a woman 20 weeks pregnant was by definition not carrying a viable fetus (according to the medical standards of the time), and that requiring her and her doctor to go through a series of tests was less about protecting a potentially viable fetus than about harassing a woman and her doctor as they pursued the perfectly legal option of a second-trimester abortion.

Thus, there were three major legal issues in *Webster:*

1. Could the state of Missouri determine that life began at conception and write such a determination into law?
2. Was it constitutional to restrict the use of public funds for abortions and for counseling that included mention of abortions, given that poor women's access to a legal medical procedure would thereby be restricted?
3. Was it constitutional to require physicians to perform certain tests on women at least 20 weeks pregnant who sought abortions, even if standard medical practice did not advise performing those tests?

Decision

In a 5–4 decision, the Court decided to overrule the lower courts and uphold much of the Missouri statute, though it unanimously declined to address the question of how public *funds* could be used. The Court did rule that public *facilities* could be barred from providing abortion. Chief Justice William Rehnquist wrote the decision for the majority, with Justices Sandra Day O'Connor and Antonin Scalia writing concurring opinions, and with Justices Byron White and Anthony Kennedy concurring. Justices William Brennan, Thurgood Marshall, Harry Blackmun, and John Paul Stevens dissented.

Rehnquist argued that the statute's preamble, holding that life begins at conception, did not specifically regulate abortion or any other medical practice; therefore, it could not violate the Constitution.

As for the question of public facilities, Rehnquist quoted an earlier court decision stating that despite the Fourteenth Amendment's guarantee of equal access to due process under the law, this did not confer an "affirmative right to governmental aid, even where such aid may be necessary to secure life, liberty, or property interests of which the government itself may not deprive the individual." In other words, the government had no right to forbid women to have early-term abortions. But neither did the government have any obligation to make such abortions equally available through the use of public facilities. If the government wanted to subsidize childbirth but not abortion, that did not constitute a violation of the Constitution, in Rehnquist's view.

Rehnquist quoted several other Supreme Court decisions to affirm that the State was indeed allowed to make value judgments concerning abortion. "Nor . . . do private physicians and their patients have some kind of constitutional right of access to public facilities for the performance of abortions," he wrote.

With regard to the issue of fetal viability and testing, Rehnquist argued that the lower courts had simply misunderstood the law. (In legal language, he said that they had "fallen into plain error.") While they read the law to mean that doctors must perform certain tests—even if those tests would not be required by standard medical practice—he read the law to say that doctors *might* perform certain tests.

Rehnquist acknowledged that fetuses at 20 weeks of age were by definition not viable, but he argued that a fetus believed to be 20 weeks old might in fact be $23^1/_2$ or 24 weeks old, and thus be potentially viable. In his argument, he cited *Roe v. Wade* itself, which recognized the State's "important and legitimate" interests in protecting the mother's health and safeguarding the potential human life of the fetus. Even *Roe*, Rehnquist argued, had found that once a fetus was viable, the State "'may, if it chooses, regulate, and even proscribe abortion except where it is necessary, in appropriate medical judgment, for the preservation of the life or health of the mother.'"

Rehnquist went on to criticize *Roe* even as he insisted that he was not overturning it. First, he wrote, *Roe* had set up a concept of trimesters—no regulation in the first; regulation regarding women's health in the second; regulation regarding fetal life in the third—that was more like a "code of regulations" than a constitutional ruling. Rehnquist quoted Justice Byron White, who had complained that the trimester framework turned the Supreme Court in the country's "*ex officio* medical board."

Besides, Rehnquist wrote, "we do not see why the State's interest in protecting potential human life should come into existence only at the point of viability . . ." Why shouldn't the State protect the fetus even before it was viable? Here Rehnquist did seem to be criticizing *Roe*, which had explicitly said that the state's interest in protecting the fetus began only when that fetus was viable. Rehnquist, by contrast, argued against "a rigid line allowing state regulation after viability but prohibiting it before viability . . . "

Rehnquist acknowledged that requiring tests of viability for women seeking abortions at 20 weeks or more of pregnancy was in effect a kind of regulation on second-trimester abortions. Again, *Roe* had said that the only permissible regulation of second-trimester abortions was to protect the health of the mother—not to protect the health of the fetus. Nevertheless, Rehnquist wrote, "we are satisfied that the requirement of these tests permissibly furthers the State's interest in protecting human life . . ." and was therefore constitutional.

Rehnquist noted that Justice Harry Blackmun, who had written a dissenting decision (and who was the majority author for *Roe*), had accused the majority "of cowardice and illegitimacy in dealing with 'the most politically divisive domestic legal issue of our time.'" Blackmun argued that the state legislatures would treat *Webster* as an invitation to restrict access to abortions. Rehnquist pointed out that more than half the U.S. population was women and expressed his confidence that the state legislatures would not "treat our decision today as an invitation to enact abortion regulation reminiscent of the dark ages."

Rehnquist ended his decision with a further affirmation that he had not intended to overturn *Roe*, even though both the U.S. Attorney General (in an *amicus* brief) and the Missouri Attorney General had asked him to do so. However, he did acknowledge that he would "modify and narrow *Roe* . . ." as his opinion had made clear.

Justice Sandra Day O'Connor wrote a concurring opinion repeating Rehnquist's claim that the Court had not overturned *Roe*. She also argued that the required tests did not "impose an undue burden on a woman's abortion decision. . . . [and] would only marginally, if at all, increase the cost of an abortion . . ."

Justice Antonin Scalia went even further in his concurring opinion: "I share Justice Blackmun's view that [this judgment] would overrule *Roe v. Wade*. I think that should be done, but would do it more explicitly." Scalia expressed his strong displeasure that the Court had contrived "to avoid almost any decision of national import." Finessing on *Roe*, he asserted, "preserves a chaos that is evident to anyone who can read and count." Abortion was a political issue, not a legal one, argued Scalia. The people's elected representatives should decide how to regulate abortion, not the lifetime appointees on the Supreme Court. To act as the Court had done today was the least responsible course that might have been chosen. Thus, Scalia wrote, "I concur in the judgment of the Court and strongly dissent from the manner which it has been reached."

Justice Harry Blackmun, who had written the majority opinion in *Roe v. Wade*, wrote the minority opinion in *Webster*, joined by Justices Brennan and

Marshall. He used strong language to describe the dangers that he believed this decision had posed to a woman's right to choose:

Today, Roe v. Wade *and the fundamental constitutional right of women to decide whether to terminate a pregnancy, survive but are not secure. . . . [T]he plurality and Justice Scalia would overrule* Roe *(the first silently, the other explicitly) and would return to the States virtually unfettered authority to control the quintessentially intimate, personal, and life-directing decision whether to carry a fetus to term. . . . [A] plurality of this Court implicitly invites every state legislature to enact more and more restrictive abortion regulations in order to provoke more and more test cases, in the hope that sometime down the line the court will return the law of procreative freedom to the severe limitations that generally prevailed in this country before January 22, 1973* [the date of *Roe v. Wade*].

Blackmun said that he could never remember when a Court had acted "in such a deceptive fashion." Rehnquist's assertion that *Roe* had been left "undisturbed," albeit "modif[ied] and narrow[ed]" was "totally meaningless," Blackmun wrote, given that this decision "filled with winks, and nods, and knowing glances" had "turn[ed] a stone face to anyone in search of . . . a women's right . . . to terminate a pregnancy free from the coercive and brooding influence of the State."

"I fear for the future," Blackmun wrote. "I fear for the liberty and equality of the millions of women who have lived and come of age in the 16 years since *Roe* was decided. I fear for the integrity of, and public esteem for, this Court."

Blackmun focused his criticisms on the viability-testing requirement, which he felt was "a radical reversal of the law of abortion." He argued that, contrary to the plurality opinion, the statute in question did indeed require doctors to perform a range of tests, whether or not those doctors thought the tests were reasonable or necessary. These tests, Blackmun argued, "impose significant additional health risks on both the pregnant woman and the fetus, and bear no rational relation to the State's interest in protecting fetal life. . . . [The provision] is an arbitrary imposition of discomfort, risk, and expense, furthering no discernible interest except to make the procurement of an abortion as arduous and difficult as possible."

"Thus," Blackmun wrote, "'not with a bang, but a whimper,' the plurality discards a landmark case of the last generation, and casts into darkness the hopes and visions of every woman in this country who had come to believe that the Constitution guaranteed her right to exercise some control over her unique ability to bear children." Blackmun mentioned the prospect of women, "especially poor and minority women," dying or being injured as they defied the law and "place[d] their health and safety in the unclean and unsympathetic hands of back-alley abortionists, or [attempted] to perform abortions upon themselves, with disastrous results . . . all in the name of enforced morality or religious dictates or lack of compassion, as it may be."

Justice John Paul Stevens also wrote a minority opinion, focusing on the preamble to the Missouri law, which had found that life began at conception, defined as "'the fertilization of the ovum of a female by a sperm of a male.'" However, Stevens wrote, standard medical texts defined "conception" as implantation in the uterus, which occurred six days after fertilization. Stevens felt that this preamble violated the separation of church and state, since the legislature had chosen an apparently religious theory of life—beginning at fertilization—rather than the prevailing medical one—beginning six days at implantation.

Therefore, Stevens wrote, the preamble "serves no identifiable secular purpose," and might infringe not only upon women's right to early-term abortions, but on their rights to methods of conception, like the IUD or the morning-after pill, which prevented fertilized eggs from being implanted. "As a secular matter," Stevens wrote, "there is an obvious difference between the state interest in protecting the freshly fertilized egg and the state interest in protecting a 9-month-gestated, fully sentient fetus on the eve of birth." As a religious matter, Stevens conceded, some might argue that the fertilized egg had a soul and thus a right to life, but as a secular matter, there was no basis for coming to this conclusion.

Impact

Webster is generally regarded by both pro-choice and pro-life advocates as a landmark decision establishing the rights of states to limit access to abortion in various ways. Although there had been a series of cases concerning this issue in the 16 years between *Roe* and *Webster,* and though the 1977 Hyde Amendment had enacted a major restriction on poor women's access to abortion (see chapter 1), the Court had repeatedly turned to *Roe* to set the parameters for how abortion might be regulated: no regulation in the first trimester; regulations concerning women's health starting in the second trimester; regulations concerning the fetus in the third trimester. Although the majority insisted that it had not overturned *Roe, Webster* was generally viewed as helping to legitimize the notion of fetal rights, opening the door to state legislatures that wanted to protect the fetus far earlier than the third trimester specified in *Roe.*

It was also significant that *Webster* allowed the government to forbid even the mention of abortion as an option in any public health facilities (except when the life of the woman was in danger). The notion that the government could use its funding and influence to discourage abortion, even if the practice was technically legal, was a major victory for the right-to-life view that saw abortion as a legal but undesirable evil—comparable, say, to drinking, or gambling—rather than a legitimate medical procedure that any woman might choose based on her own conscience and desires. The notion that the government could treat abortion as undesirable, rather than as one medical option among many, was a major shift from the climate of the early 1970s in which *Roe* had been decided.

PLANNED PARENTHOOD OF SOUTHEASTERN PENNSYLVANIA V. CASEY (1992)

Background

In 1989, the state of Pennsylvania passed the Abortion Control Act, a statute with several provisions regulating abortion in various ways. Except in narrowly defined medical emergencies,

1) A woman must wait 24 hours between consenting to an abortion and receiving one.
2) At least 24 hours before performing an abortion, a physician must inform the woman of the nature of the procedure, the health risks of the abortion, and the "probable gestational age of the unborn child," and a qualified person must inform the woman of the availability of state-mandated printed materials describing the fetus and providing information about medical assistance for childbirth, information about child support from the father, and a list of agencies that provide adoption and other services as alternatives to abortion. The woman must certify in writing that she has been told about these materials and given the chance to view them.
3) A married woman must provide a signed statement that her husband has been told of her intention to have an abortion or else she must provide a signed statement that her husband is not the man who impregnated her; that the husband could not be located; that the pregnancy was the result of a sexual assault by the husband that she had reported; or that she believes that notifying her husband will cause him or someone else to inflict bodily injury upon her. Any doctor who performed an abortion without one of these signed statements would have his or her license revoked and would be liable to the husband for damages.
4) A minor cannot receive an abortion without the consent, provided in person at the clinic, of a parent or guardian, except when a judge has waived this provision.

Reproductive Rights and Technology

In addition, doctors and clinics that performed abortions were required to provide the state with annual statistical reports on procedures performed during the year, including the names of doctors.

These provisions of the law were challenged by five abortion clinics, a doctor representing himself, and a class of doctors who provide abortion. The plaintiffs charged that this law was unconstitutional. The Federal District Court entered first a preliminary and then a permanent injunction against enforcement of this law. The Third Circuit Court of Appeals reversed the lower court's decision, finding that the law was constitutional except for the provision requiring husbands to be notified. The Supreme Court agreed to hear the appeal.

As is usual in major cases, the Court received several "friend of the Court" briefs—documents from interested parties who were trying to influence its decision with their own legal arguments. One such brief was from the U.S. government (under President George H. W. Bush), asking the Court to overturn *Roe v. Wade*, its landmark 1973 decision that had established a woman's fundamental right to an abortion.

Legal Issues

There were two major legal issues in *Planned Parenthood v. Casey:* first, should the Court uphold *Roe v. Wade;* and, second, in what ways might a state regulate abortions?

Roe had been the subject of controversy ever since it was rendered in 1973, and for several years, many Supreme Court Justices had proclaimed it to be a bad decision. Justice Scalia, in particular, had argued that by forbidding legislators to regulate abortion, *Roe* was profoundly undemocratic. The ones who should make decisions regarding abortions, Scalia argued, were the democratically elected representatives of the people, not the lifetime appointees on the Supreme Court. Justice Byron White had written the minority opinion in *Roe*, while both Chief Justice William Rehnquist and Justice Clarence Thomas were well-known *Roe* opponents.

On the other hand, overturning a prior Supreme Court decision was no light matter. Much of the language in *Casey*, in fact, concerned the seriousness of such an action, and the Court's belief that overturning prior decisions tended to undermine the credibility and prestige of the Court. Whether or not individual Justices would have supported *Roe* had they been on the Court in 1973, was a separate issue from whether they had the right or the duty to overturn it now.

With regard to abortion regulations, the Court had already struck down informed-consent provisions in *Thornburgh v. American College of Obstetricians and Gynecologists* (1986), which also involved Pennsylvania law. In *Thorn-

burgh, the Court had argued that such provisions were intended not to inform women at all but rather to persuade them not to have abortions, thus interfering with their rights to privacy under *Roe v. Wade*.

Concerning the notification of minors' parents, the Court had ruled in *Ohio v. Akron Center for Reproductive Health* (1990) that a doctor performing an abortion on a minor had to personally notify her parent or guardian 24 hours before the procedure. In that case, the Court had ruled that as long as judicial bypass was available, the law was constitutional.

Since *Thornburgh*, several pro-life Justices had been appointed to the Court. Thus activists on both sides of the abortion issue watched eagerly to see whether the Court would continue to uphold *Roe*, and what kinds of abortion regulation it would find permissible.

Decision

The Court ruled 5–4 to uphold *Roe*. However, the majority decision by Justices O'Connor, Kennedy, and Souter offered a radical redefinition of *Roe*. Previously, *Roe* had been seen as upholding a woman's fundamental right to choose abortion. Thus, any interference with that right was generally viewed as unconstitutional. However, *Roe* did provide for regulation of abortion to protect a woman's health beginning in the second trimester; and regulation to protect the potential life of the fetus after viability, which was then considered to begin in the third trimester.

Casey threw out the trimester system and asserted instead that the State had a compelling interest in protecting the fetus from "the outset of the pregnancy." Therefore, rather than seeing abortion as a "fundamental" right, the Court would construct a new standard: Restrictions on abortion would be allowed as long as they did not constitute an "undue burden" on the woman's right to choose. Therefore, a state could try to discourage a woman from choosing abortion, as long as its actions did not create an "undue obstacle" to her right to choose. Certain obstacles were permitted—but they could not be "undue" obstacles.

With this approach, requiring a woman to view pictures of a fetus before having an abortion might not be considered an "undue burden," as she would still be free to choose the procedure after viewing the pictures. Requiring a woman to tell her husband about an abortion, on the other hand, might very well constitute an undue burden, since any woman who feared psychological or physical abuse from her husband might be unable to have an abortion for that reason.

Using "undue burden" as its new criterion, the Court upheld the Pennsylvania law's 24-hour waiting period; its requirement that a woman be given state-mandated information on abortion and offered state-authored materials on fetal development; and its requirement that a minor's parent or guardian give consent to the doctor in person. The Court also found that the requirement of providing abortion statistics could be viewed as research in the interests of public health, and so it was ruled constitutional.

The Court spoke directly to critics who had argued that a 24-hour waiting period would in fact prevent many women from choosing abortions, because "for those who have the fewest financial resources, those who must travel long distances, and those who have difficulty explaining their whereabouts to husbands, empoyers, or others, the 24-hour waiting period will be 'particularly burdensome.'"

The court replied:

These findings are troubling in some respects, but they do not demonstrate that the waiting period constitutes an undue burden. . . . [U]nder the undue burden standard a State is permitted to enact persuasive measures which favor childbirth over abortion, even if those measures do not further a health interest. And while the waiting period does limit a physician's discretion, that is not, standing alone, a reason to invalidate it.

The Court did decide, however, that laws involving a woman's husband in an abortion decision were an undue burden, and they therefore struck down that provision.

Objecting strongly to much of this decision was Justice Harry Blackmun, the original author of *Roe*. Blackmun wrote passionately of the women who would be compelled to carry unwanted pregnancies to term as a result of the restrictions allowed by this decision, and he introduced a personal note into his fears: "I am 83 years old. I cannot remain on this Court forever, and when I do step down, the confirmation process for my successor well may focus on the issue before us today."

Justice Stevens seemed to accept the notion of "undue burden," but to disagree with the way the plurality had chosen to apply it. "A burden may be 'undue,'" he wrote, "either because the burden is too severe or because it lacks a legitimate, rational justification. The 24-hour delay requirement fails both parts of this test."

Like Blackmun, Stevens also objected to the requirement that a woman be provided with certain information. Because such information served no useful purpose, he wrote, it therefore "constitute[d] an undue burden on the woman's constitutional liberty to decide to terminate her pregnancy." The reporting requirement, Stevens added, served no useful public health purpose and should be struck down.

Writing for the minority, Chief Justice William Rehnquist argued strongly for the overturning of *Roe v. Wade* and for upholding the entire

Pennsylvania law. He called the undue burden standard "an unjustified constitutional compromise, one which leaves the Court in a position to scrutinize all types of abortion regulations despite the fact that it lacks the power to do so under the Constitution."

Rehnquist reiterated the major objections to *Roe:* that because abortion "involves the purposeful termination of potential life," it is a special kind of right, "different in kind from the others that the Court has protected under the rubric of personal or family privacy or autonomy"; that the historical traditions of the American people do not support the view that the right to terminate a pregnancy is "fundamental"; and that the "abortion code" imposed by *Roe* was far too specific for a Constitution that spoke in only "general terms."

Scalia, too, repeated his opposition to *Roe.* Just because the Court had once made a mistake, he argued, was no reason not to correct it:

> *I cannot agree with, indeed I am appalled by, the court's suggestion that the decision to stand by an erroneous constitutional decision must be strongly influenced—against overruling, no less—by the substantial and continuing public opposition the decision has generated. The Court's judgment that any other course would "subvert the Court's legitimacy" must be another consequence of reading the error-filled history book that described the deeply divided country brought together by* Roe.

Impact

The full impact of *Casey* has yet to be determined, for one of the major legacies of this decision was the possibility that the Supreme Court might overturn *Roe.* Certainly, this question was a major issue in the 2000 presidential elections. Although the newly elected president George W. Bush and his Attorney General John Ashcroft have pledged to support *Roe,* pro-choice activists cite *Casey* as a reason to worry: Even if *Roe* is upheld in theory, they argue, its guarantees will be moot in practice, particularly for low-income women and teenagers, as numerous regulations make abortions de facto out of reach for many women.

Pro-life activists, on the other hand, had a divided reaction to *Casey.* On the one hand, they saw the possibility of passing restrictive state laws, as had been done in Pennsylvania—laws that would no longer be overturned by the Supreme Court. On the other hand, they continued to be offended by the notion that, in principle, the choice for abortion was a private one that each woman had the right to make for herself, rather than a public matter of society protecting the unborn.

DON STENBERG, ATTORNEY GENERAL OF NEBRASKA, ET AL. PETITIONERS V. LEROY CARHART (2000)

Background

The state of Nebraska passed a law banning a procedure that it termed "partial-birth abortion," a colloquial term whose exact meaning became the subject of legal controversy. The law was challenged by Dr. Leroy Carhart, a Nebraska physician who performs abortions in a clinical setting. Carhart went to federal district court asking for a declaration that the Nebraska statute violated the federal Constitution and seeking an injunction forbidding its enforcement. During the trial, both sides called expert witnesses to explain the various medical procedures involved in performing different types of abortions and to discuss the question of which abortion procedures might be safer in various circumstances. The District Court found the law unconstitutional, an opinion affirmed by the Eighth Circuit Court of Appeals. The Supreme Court agreed to consider the case.

Legal Issues

Stenberg v. Carhart is unusual among Supreme Court cases on abortion for the large amount of medical detail included in the opinions, including graphic descriptions of various abortion procedures. This is because one of the major legal issues in the case concerned exactly which procedures were banned under the law. Another major issue was the relative safety of various procedures, and the extent to which a particular procedure might be needed by a particular woman.

There were three major legal issues in this case:

1) *What exactly is a "partial-birth abortion"?* Did the Nebraska law prevent only the abortion known as D&X (dilation and extraction), a relatively rare procedure, or might it also apply to D&E (dilation and evacuation), a fairly common procedure used in most second-trimester abortions?

2) *Was it acceptable that the Nebraska law offered no exceptions to its ban in order to safeguard a woman's health?* The law did allow "partial-birth" abortions to be performed to "save the life of the mother"—but not to protect her health.

3) *Did this ban on "partial-birth abortion" constitute an "undue burden" on a woman's ability to exercise her right to an abortion?* Since the law might be interpreted to ban the commonly used procedure known as

D&E, was that making it unduly difficult for a woman to exercise her right to choose?

Decision

The Supreme Court, in a 5–4 vote, agreed with the lower court decisions and struck down the Nebraska law. Justice Stephen Breyer, writing for the majority, reaffirmed the principle established in *Roe v. Wade*, "that the Constitution offers basic protection to the woman's right to choose." He explained that this decision was based on the three principles that had already been established in *Planned Parenthood v. Casey:*

1) Before a fetus is viable, a woman has the right to choose to end her pregnancy.
2) A law designed to protect the life of a viable fetus could not at the same time impose "an undue burden" on the woman seeking an abortion before viability. Any law intended to protect the viable fetus also had to protect a woman's right to abort a nonviable fetus.
3) The state was allowed to regulate and even ban abortions that might threaten the life of a viable fetus, but it always had to include an exception for abortions that were "necessary, in appropriate medical judgment, for the preservation of the life or health of the mother." The Nebraska law did not include such an exception; hence, it was unconstitutional.

Breyer quoted extensively from the opinions of various doctors and medical organizations to show that the D&X procedure might indeed be the best one for a woman's health under certain circumstances. He found no reason to restrict women from this option, if it was indeed better for their health.

Moreover, he wrote, the law might be used to ban D&E procedures, as well as D&X procedures. Since D&E procedures were so commonly used for second-trimester abortions, banning them would indeed constitute an "undue burden" upon a woman's right to have an abortion.

Justice Antonin Scalia, in his dissent, repeated his ongoing assertion that the Supreme Court ought not to be deciding on such controversial matters as abortion but should rather leave that issue to the people to decide through their elected representatives. He called for the overturn of the *Casey* decision, taking issue with the notion of "undue burden," which he had written then was "hopelessly unworkable in practice" and "ultimately standardless." Moreover, he personally found the type of abortion banned in Nebraska "so horrible that the most clinical description of it evokes a shudder of revulsion." Scalia also argued that allowing for a "health exception" pronounced by "the abortionist . . . himself . . . [sic] is to give live-birth abortion free rein."

Justice Clarence Thomas, joined by Scalia and Chief Justice Rehnquist, repeated his and his colleagues' opposition to *Roe v. Wade* itself, as well as to the practice of abortion. "Abortion," he wrote, 'is a unique act, in which a woman's exercise of control over her own body ends, depending on one's view, human life or potential human life. Nothing in our Federal Constitution deprives the people of this country of the right to determine whether the consequences of abortion to the fetus and to society outweight the burden of an unwanted pregnancy on the mother."

Like Scalia, Thomas also expressed his opposition to the *Casey* decision, which he felt "was constructed by its authors out of whole cloth." And, like Scalia, he expressed his revulsion at the particular form of abortion banned by Nebraska, which he called "so gruesome that its use can be traumatic even for the physicians and medical staff who perform it." Indeed, he wrote, the method "so closely borders on infanticide that 30 states have attempted to ban it."

Thomas objected to what he considered Breyer's "sanitized description" of the abortion procedures involved, and provided his own more graphic and emotional account, based on the testimony of a nurse who had observed a "partial-birth abortion." She described "[t]he baby's little fingers" and "little feet," speaking of the fetus's reaction as "like a startle reaction, like a flinch, like a baby does when he thinks he is going to fall."

"The question whether States have a legitimate interest in banning the procedure does not require additional authority," wrote Thomas. "In a civilized society, the answer is too obvious, and the contrary arguments too offensive to merit further discussion."

Impact

The impact of *Stenberg v. Carhart* is still being decided and will no doubt depend greatly on the Supreme Court appointments that fall to the authority of President George W. Bush. Both pro-life and pro-choice forces were well aware that *Stenberg* was decided by a 5–4 vote, and that the appointment of even one new Supreme Court Justice who opposed *Roe* would likely tip the balance of the Court. Even though *Stenberg* itself upheld both *Roe* and *Casey*, the number of justices who expressed their disapproval of these decisions, and the vehemence they displayed, made it clear that the sentiment on the Court had shifted greatly since *Roe* was decided in 1973.

On the other hand, the decision was considered a pro-choice victory, as it did strike down a law that restricted abortion methods, and as it made the term *partial-birth abortion* more difficult to use in a legal context. Supporters of abortion rights object to the term *partial-birth abortion* as vague, misleading, and inflammatory. Opponents of abortion argue that the term is more honest and direct than medical language such as "dilation and extraction" or "dilation and evacuation."

The decision was also a pro-choice victory in that it emphasized that the woman's health took precedence over the fetus's rights—even over the rights of a viable fetus. This approach stands in stark contrast to the attitudes expressed in the "Unborn Victims of Violence Act," a 1999 measure passed overwhelmingly by the House of Representatives affirming that the rights of "unborn children," beginning at conception, are equal to and separate from the rights of the women who carried them. This is a position that is gaining ground in the United States, but *Stenberg* made it clear that such an attitude had not yet been affirmed by the members of the Supreme Court.

SUMMARY OF STATE LAWS AND REGULATIONS REGARDING ABORTION AND CONTRACEPTION

State Constitutional Rulings

In 18 states, courts have ruled that their state constitutions provide greater protection for women's right to choose reproductive options than the federal constitution: Alaska, Arizona, California, Connecticut, Florida, Idaho, Illinois, Indiana, Massachusetts, Minnesota, Montana, New Jersey, New Mexico, Oregon, Tennessee, Texas, Vermont, and West Virginia.

The U.S. Supreme Court has ruled that it is constitutional to ban medically necessary abortions from medical assistance programs. However, in 16 states, courts have ruled that their state constitutions prohibit such exclusion: Alaska, Arizona, California, Connecticut, Idaho, Illinois, Indiana, Massachusetts, Minnesota, Montana, New Jersey, New Mexico, Oregon, Texas, Vermont, and West Virginia. In six states—California, Massachusetts, Minnesota, New Jersey, New Mexico, and West Virginia—the ruling was by the state's highest court.

Five state courts—in Alaska, California, Florida, Montana, and New Jersey—have ruled that the state constitution does not allow laws requiring parental consent or notice for minors having abortions. Although Massachusetts's legislature passed a law requiring a minor to get both parents' consent for an abortion, the state's highest court ruled that the law violates the state's Declaration of Rights (constitution), even with a judicial bypass, and has ordered that the law be enforced as if it required the consent of only one parent. The U.S. Supreme Court, however, has held it is constitutional to require two-parent notice, as long as judicial bypass is available. (Judicial bypass is a provision that allows a judge to permit exceptions to the law. When a parent cannot be located, is not competent to make a decision for a minor, or might abuse a minor, a judge might rule that the parent does not have to be informed.)

The Supreme Court has ruled that the U.S. Constitution permits states to require a waiting period and to mandate that certain information be provided to women seeking abortion. But some state courts have ruled that their state constitutions do not allow such requirements. A state court in Montana has ruled against a 24-hour waiting period, while Tennessee's highest court has found against a 3-day waiting period. Nor is it permissible in either state to require abortion providers to give state-mandated information about abortion to women.

The Alaska Supreme Court has found that "conscience-based exemptions" (allowing personnel or institutions to refuse to participate in abortion on the basis of moral or religious beliefs) are not allowable under the state constitution when they apply to "quasi-public" institutions. The U.S. Supreme Court has upheld another Alaska law that bars abortion from public facilities.

A Montana court has found that the state constitution will not allow provisions barring physicians' assistants from performing abortions. (A physician's assistant is a trained medical staff person who performs many of the duties once reserved only for doctors.)

Some State Statutes and Regulations Concerning Abortion

Abortion Bans, pre-*Roe* Fifteen states and the District of Columbia have not repealed their pre-*Roe* bans on abortion, even though, under *Roe*, these are unconstitutional and unenforceable: Alabama, Arizona, Arkansas, California, Colorado, Delaware, Washington, D.C., Massachusetts, Michigan, Mississippi, New Mexico, Oklahoma, Texas, Vermont, West Virginia, and Wisconsin.

Abortion Bans, post-*Roe* After the 1989 Supreme Court decision, *Webster v. Reproductive Health Services* (see above), Louisiana and Utah enacted unenforceable laws banning most abortions. Louisiana law forbids abortion except if the woman's life is endangered or in the case of rape or incest. Utah law prohibits abortion before 20 weeks except when the woman's life or health are in danger; in the case of reported rape or incest; or if there are serious fetal anomalies. Abortions after 20 weeks are banned except when the woman's life or health are in danger or in the case of serious fetal anomalies. These laws have been ruled unconstitutional.

Bans on Abortion Procedures Thirty-one states have passed laws that ban particular abortion procedures: Alabama, Alaska, Arizona, Arkansas, Florida, Georgia, Idaho, Illinois, Indiana, Iowa, Kansas, Kentucky, Louisiana, Michigan, Mississippi, Missouri, Montana, Nebraska, New Jersey, New Mexico, North Dakota, Ohio, Oklahoma, Rhode Island, South Carolina, South Dakota, Tennessee, Utah, Virginia, West Virginia, and Wisconsin.

In 2000, in *Stenberg v. Carhart* (see above), the U.S. Supreme Court ruled that Nebraska's ban on "partial-birth abortion" was unconstitutional. The Nebraska law bans more than one procedure and lacks any exception to protect a woman's health. Both because of *Stenberg* and because of other lawsuits, bans on "partial-birth abortions" and other procedures are unconstitutional and unenforceable in at least 29 states: Alabama, Alaska, Arizona, Arkansas, Florida, Idaho, Illinois, Indiana, Iowa, Kansas, Kentucky, Louisiana, Michigan, Mississippi, Missouri, Montana, Nebraska, New Jersey, New Mexico, North Dakota, Ohio, Oklahoma, Rhode Island, South Carolina, South Dakota, Tennessee, Virginia, West Virginia, and Wisconsin.

Clinic Violence and Harassment Fourteen states and the District of Columbia have passed laws to protect both clinic personnel and women seeking services from blocked access to clinics and violence: California, Colorado, Washington, D.C., Kansas, Maine, Maryland, Massachusetts, Michigan, Minnesota, Nevada, New York, North Carolina, Oregon, Washington, and Wisconsin. In 2000, the U.S. Supreme Court upheld a Colorado law that established a "no-approach zone" intended to protect patients and clinics from violence and harassment. On the other hand, a court preliminarily enjoined enforcement of the "bubble zone" law in Massachusetts, which had the same intention.

Conscience-based Exemptions Forty-five states allow some medical staff and institutions to refuse to participate in abortion on the basis of moral or religious beliefs: Alaska, Arizona, Arkansas, California, Colorado, Connecticut, Delaware, Florida, Georgia, Hawaii, Idaho, Illinois, Indiana, Iowa, Kansas, Kentucky, Louisiana, Maine, Maryland, Massachusetts, Michigan, Minnesota, Missouri, Montana, Nebraska, Nevada, New Jersey, New Mexico, New York, North Carolina, North Dakota, Ohio, Oklahoma, Oregon, Pennsylvania, Rhode Island, South Carolina, South Dakota, Tennessee, Texas, Utah, Virginia, Washington, Wisconsin, and Wyoming. In Alaska, Minnesota, and New Jersey, courts have ruled that such laws are unconstitutional when they are applied to public, "quasi-public," nonsectarian, and/or nonprofit institutions.

South Dakota has a law allowing pharmacists to refuse to dispense medication if there is reason to believe that the medication will be used to induce abortion.

West Virginia allows medical personnel to refuse to perform an abortion on a minor.

Counseling Bans Fifteen states have "gag rules" prohibiting certain state employees or state-funded groups from mentioning abortion as a possibility in counseling women and/or from referring women to abortion services under certain circumstances: Arizona, Illinois, Indiana, Kentucky, Louisiana, Michigan, Minnesota, Mississippi, Missouri, Nebraska, North Dakota, Ohio, Pennsylvania, Virginia, and Wisconsin. Kentucky law bans emergency room personnel who are treating sexually assaulted women from mentioning abortion or making referrals.

North Dakota's law, which bans any group that makes abortion referrals from receiving state family planning funds, has been held unconstitutional.

Husband Consent and Notice Nine states have unenforceable laws requiring the husbands of married women to be notified or to give their consent before their wives may have abortions: Colorado, Illinois, Kentucky, Louisiana, North Dakota, Pennsylvania, Rhode Island, South Carolina, and Utah. These laws are unenforceable because of *Planned Parenthood v. Casey*, the U.S. Supreme Court ruling that found it unconstitutional to require a husband's notification or consent.

"Informed Consent" and Waiting Periods Informed consent laws generally require that women be given certain information before being allowed to have abortions, such as state-mandated lectures or reading material on fetal development; facts about support services for continuing the pregnancy; and information about adoption. Thirty states have abortion-specific "informed consent" laws: Alabama, Alaska, California, Connecticut, Delaware, Florida, Idaho, Indiana, Kansas, Kentucky, Louisiana, Maine, Massachusetts, Michigan, Minnesota, Mississippi, Missouri, Montana, Nebraska, Nevada, North Dakota, Ohio, Pennsylvania, Rhode Island, South Carolina, South Dakota, Tennessee, Utah, Virginia, and Wisconsin. A Florida court has issued a temporary injunction prohibiting enforcement of such a law. Missouri and Tennessee courts have found such laws unconstitutional. A Montana court has issued a permanent injunction against enforcement of such a law.

Nineteen states require waiting periods to begin after a woman receives either a state-mandated lecture or reading materials: Delaware,

Idaho, Indiana, Kansas, Kentucky, Louisiana, Massachusetts, Michigan, Mississippi, Montana, Nebraska, North Dakota, Ohio, Pennsylvania, South Carolina, South Dakota, Tennessee, Utah, and Wisconsin. The waiting period is actually enforced in fifteen of these states: Idaho, Indiana, Kansas, Kentucky, Louisiana, Michigan, Mississippi, Nebraska, North Dakota, Ohio, Pennsylvania, South Carolina, South Dakota, Utah, and Wisconsin.

Insurance Six states will not allow private insurance coverage for abortion unless the woman pays a higher premium: Idaho, Kentucky, Missouri, North Dakota, Rhode Island, and Wisconsin. However, in Wisconsin, the law applies only to a particular voluntary program for private employers known as the Private Employer Health Care Purchasing Alliance.

Courts have found the Rhode Island law to be unconstitutional. Pennsylvania law requires insurers to offer a policy alternative that excludes abortion. Massachusetts law specifies that HMOs do not have to pay for abortions or make referrals to abortion providers.

Eleven states specify that public funds may not be used to pay for insurance that includes abortion coverage: Arkansas, Colorado, Illinois, Kentucky, Massachusetts, Michigan, Nebraska, Ohio, Pennsylvania, Rhode Island, and Virginia. Massachusetts law also says that health insurance purchased for state employees may not cover so-called partial-birth abortions performed after the fetus is viable. The Rhode Island law has been ruled unconstitutional in its application to city employees. Michigan, Nebraska, and Ohio law allows some public health employees to buy a rider for health care coverage for abortion services.

Legislative Declarations Ten state legislatures have passed laws declaring their intention of protecting the life of the "unborn": Arkansas, Illinois, Kentucky, Louisiana, Missouri, Montana, Nebraska, North Dakota, Pennsylvania, and Utah.

Five state legislatures have passed laws declaring their support for a woman's right to choose abortion: Connecticut, Maine, Maryland, Nevada, and Washington. The Nevada law, which protects a woman's right to choose during the first 24 weeks of pregnancy, cannot be changed except by referendum.

Physician-Only Requirements Forty-four states have laws requiring that only a doctor may perform an abortion: Alabama, Alaska, Arkansas, California, Colorado, Connecticut, Delaware, Florida, Georgia, Hawaii,

Idaho, Illinois, Indiana, Iowa, Kentucky, Louisiana, Maine, Maryland, Massachusetts, Michigan, Minnesota, Mississippi, Missouri, Montana, Nebraska, Nevada, New Jersey, New Mexico, New York, North Carolina, North Dakota, Ohio, Oklahoma, Pennsylvania, Rhode Island, South Carolina, South Dakota, Tennessee, Texas, Utah, Virginia, Washington, Wisconsin, and Wyoming. However, there may also be other laws, regulations, or provisions in those states that allow non-physician clinicians to perform abortions.

Montana's law, which prohibited physician assistants from performing abortions, has been permanently enjoined by a court.

The Rhode Island law allows either a doctor or a licensed health care practitioner acting within the scope of his or her practice to perform abortions; however, only a doctor may perform surgical abortions.

In Kentucky, first-trimester abortions can be performed only by a doctor, or by the woman herself upon a doctor's advice; after the first trimester, only a doctor may perform abortions.

In New York, abortions can be performed only by a doctor—or by a woman acting upon her doctor's advice that such an act is necessary to preserve her life or within 24 weeks of the start of her pregnancy.

Oklahoma law forbids any woman from inducing her own abortion, except under a doctor's supervision.

A District of Columbia law states that abortions can be performed only under the direction of a licensed practitioner of medicine.

Post-Viability Bans Forty states and the District of Columbia restrict abortion in various ways once the fetus is presumed viable: Alabama, Arizona, Arkansas, California, Connecticut, Delaware, Washington, D.C., Florida, Georgia, Idaho, Illinois, Indiana, Iowa, Kansas, Kentucky, Louisiana, Maine, Maryland, Massachusetts, Mississippi, Minnesota, Missouri, Montana, Nebraska, Nevada, New York, North Carolina, North Dakota, Ohio, Oklahoma, Pennsylvania, Rhode Island, South Carolina, South Dakota, Tennessee, Texas, Utah, Virginia, Washington, Wisconsin, and Wyoming.

Public Employees and Public Facilities Only Missouri prohibits a public employee from participating in the provision of abortion services. (See *Webster*, above.)

Eight states, however, forbid certain public facilities from providing abortions under certain circumstances: Arizona, Iowa, Kansas, Kentucky, Louisiana, Missouri, North Dakota, and Pennsylvania.

Viability Testing Five states require doctors to test fetuses for viability under certain circumstances: Alabama, Kansas, Missouri, Ohio, and Pennsylvania. In Pennsylvania, doctors have to determine viability for any abortion performed after the first trimester.

The Ohio law has been found unconstitutional by the courts, and there is a permanent injunction against its enforcement.

Two states—Arizona and Louisiana—require that a woman have ultrasound before getting an abortion. In Arizona, the ultrasound is mandatory for women seeking abortions after 12 weeks of pregnancy. In Louisiana, the law requires an ultrasound for any woman seeking abortion in order to determine the stage of pregnancy; however, a court has permanently enjoined this law.

MANDATORY WAITING PERIOD FOR ABORTION

State	Waiting Period	Enforced	Enjoined/Not Enforced
Delaware	min. 24 hours		X
Idaho	min. 24 hours	X[1]	
Indiana	min. 18 hours	X	
Kansas	min. 24 hours	X	
Kentucky	min. 24 hours	X[2]	
Louisiana	min. 24 hours	X	
Massachusetts	min. 24 hours		X[3]
Michigan	min. 24 hours	X	
Mississippi	min. 24 hours	X	
Montana	min. 24 hours		X[4]
Nebraska	min. 24 hours	X	
North Dakota	min. 24 hours	X	
Ohio	min. 24 hours	X	
Pennsylvania	min. 24 hours	X	
South Carolina	min. 1 hour	X	
Tennessee	min. 48–72 hours		X[3]
Utah	min. 24 hours	X	
Wisconsin	min. 24 hours	X	

[1] A woman must be provided with state-prepared materials at least 24 hours before an abortion, if reasonably possible.

[2] A court has ruled that this law is constitutional and has indicated that it anticipates lifting a stay of enforcement.

[3] A court has ruled that this waiting period provision is unconstitutional.

[4] This law provides that a woman may not obtain an abortion until the third day after her initial consultation.

RESTRICTIONS ON MINORS' ACCESS TO ABORTION

State	One-Parent	Two-Parent	Consent	Notice	Judicial Bypass	Enjoined/ Not Enforced	Enforced
Alabama	X		X		X		X
Alaska	X		X		X	X[1]	
Arizona	X		X		X	X[1]	
Arkansas		X		X	X		X
California	X		X		X	X[1]	
Colorado	X[11]			X		X	
Delaware	X[2]			X[3]	X		X
Florida	X			X	X	X[1]	
Georgia	X			X	X		X
Idaho	X		X[12]		X		X
Illinois	X[5]			X	X	X[1]	
Indiana	X		X		X		X
Iowa	X[2]			X	X		X
Kansas	X			X	X		X
Kentucky	X		X		X		X
Louisiana	X		X		X		X
Maine	X[6]		X[7]		X		X
Maryland	X			X[3]			X
Massachusetts	X[8]		X		X		X
Michigan	X		X		X		X
Minnesota		X		X	X		X
Mississippi		X	X		X		X
Missouri	X		X		X		X
Montana	X			X	X	X[1]	
Nebraska	X			X	X		X
Nevada	X			X	X	X[1]	
New Jersey	X			X	X	X	
New Mexico	X		X			X[1]	
North Carolina	X[2]		X		X		X
North Dakota		X	X		X		X
Ohio	X[9]			X	X		X
Pennsylvania	X		X		X		X
Rhode Island	X		X		X		X
South Carolina	X[2]		X		X		X
South Dakota	X			X	X		X
Tennessee	X		X		X		X
Texas	X			X	X		X
Utah		X[4]		X			X
Virginia	X			X	X		X
West Virginia	X			X[3]	X		X
Wisconsin	X[10]		X		X		X
Wyoming	X		X		X		X
Total	37	5	22	20	38	10	32

[1] This statute has been declared unenforceable by a court or an attorney general.

[2] This statute also allows consent or notice to a grandparent in certain circumstances.

86

3 This requirement may be waived by a specified health professional under certain circumstances.

4 This statue requires notice to a minor's parents, if possible.

5 This statute also allows consent of or notice to a grandparent or step-parent.

6 This statute also allows consent of an adult family member.

7 This statute requires mandatory counseling and allows a minor to obtain an abortion without parental consent if the doctor secures informed written consent of the minor, and if the minor is mentally and physically competent to give consent.

8 This statute requires two-parent consent, but a court has issued an order that the law be enforced as requiring the consent of only one parent.

9 This statute also allows notice to a grandparent, step-parent, or adult sibling over the age of 21 under certain circumstances.

10 This statute allows consent of or notice to a grandparent or certain other adult family members over the age of 25.

11 This statute requires notice to both parents, but allows notice to one parent, if the minor requests and if the parents do not reside together.

12 If there is a medical emergency, the physician may perform an abortion without parental consent but must attempt to notify a parent of the procedure and to obtain consent.

PUBLIC FUNDING FOR ABORTION

State	Life Endangerment	Life, Rape, Incest Only	Life, Rape, Incest, & Some Health Circumstances	All or Most Circumstances
Alabama		X		
Alaska				X[3]
Arizona				X[3]
Arkansas		X[2]		
California				X[3]
Colorado		X[2]		
Connecticut				X[3]
Delaware		X[6]		
District of Columbia		X		
Florida		X		
Georgia		X		
Hawaii				X
Idaho			X[3,6]	
Illinois			X[2,4]	
Indiana				X[3]
Iowa			X[5,6]	
Kansas		X		
Kentucky		X[2]		
Louisiana		X[2,6]		
Maine		X		
Maryland				X[5,6]
Massachusetts				X[3,6]

(continued)

PUBLIC FUNDING FOR ABORTION *(continued)*

State	Life Endangerment	Life, Rape, Incest Only	Life, Rape, Incest, & Some Health Circumstances	All or Most Circumstances
Michigan		X[2]		
Mississippi	X			
Missouri		X[2]		
Montana				X[3,6]
Nebraska		X[2]		
Nevada		X		
New Hampshire		X		
New Jersey				X[3]
New Mexico				X[3]
New York				X
North Carolina		X		
North Dakota		X[2]		
Ohio		X[6]		
Oklahoma		X[2,6]		
Oregon				X[3]
Pennsylvania		X[6]		
Rhode Island		X		
South Carolina		X[6]		
South Dakota	X			
Tennessee		X		
Texas				X[3]
Utah		X[2,6]		
Vermont				X[3]
Virginia			X[5,6]	
Washington				X
West Virginia				X[3]
Wisconsin			X[6]	
Wyoming		X[6]		
Total	2	26	5	18

Note: This chart documents official state policies for public funding and may not necessarily reflect the actual implementation of these policies.

[1] Such state policies violate federal law prohibiting participating states from excluding abortion from the Medicaid program in cases of life endangerment, rape, and incest.

[2] A court has ruled that this state must comply with federal law prohibiting the exclusion of abortion from Medicaid in cases of rape or incest as well as life endangerment.

[3] A court has ruled that the state constitution prohibits the state from restricting funding for abortion while providing funds for costs associated with childbirth or other medically necessary services.

[4] A court has ruled that the state constitution prohibits the enforcement of a state law restricting funding to the extent that it bars funding for an abortion necessary to preserve the woman's health.

[5] This statute provides funding for some cases of fetal anomaly.

[6] This state requires that cases of rape and incest be reported to a law enforcement or social service agency in some circumstances in order for the woman to be eligible for a publicly funded abortion.

The Law of Reproductive Rights and Technology

Some Statutes and Regulations Concerning Contraception

Conscience-Based Exemptions Thirty states have at least one conscience-based exemption law concerning contraception.

Twenty-five states allow some individuals and institutions to refuse to participate in giving out contraceptive supplies or services: Arkansas, Colorado, Florida, Georgia, Idaho, Illinois, Kansas, Kentucky, Maine, Maryland, Massachusetts, Minnesota, Montana, New Jersey, New Mexico, New York, North Carolina, Oregon, Pennsylvania, Rhode Island, Tennessee, Virginia, West Virginia, Wisconsin, and Wyoming.

Of these 25 states, 11 explicitly permit individuals and institutions to refuse to give patients information or counseling about contraception: Arkansas, Colorado, Florida, Georgia, Illinois, Maine, Massachusetts, Minnesota, Montana, Tennessee, and Virginia. In 10 states, individuals and institutions can refuse to give information or counseling about sterilization: Idaho, Kansas, Kentucky, Maryland, Massachusetts, Montana, New Mexico, North Carolina, Pennsylvania, and Rhode Island. In Arkansas, pharmacists are allowed by law to refuse to supply patients with contraceptive supplies. And in nine states, insurance laws concerning contraceptives allow religious employers and/or insurers to refuse to provide coverage for contraception: California, Connecticut, Delaware, Hawaii, Maine, Maryland, Nevada, North Carolina, and Rhode Island.

INSURANCE COVERAGE FOR CONTRACEPTION

State	Private Insurance		State Employees		
	Coverage Required	Coverage Not Required	Coverage Required	Coverage Not Required	Coverage Available[1]
Alabama		X		X	
Alaska		X		X	
Arizona		X		X	X
Arkansas		X		X	
California	X		X		X
Colorado	X[2]			X	X
Connecticut	X		X		X[10]
Delaware	X		X		X
District of Columbia		X		X	X
Florida		X	X		X
Georgia	X		X		X
Hawaii	X		X		X
Idaho	X[2]			X	X
Illinois		X		X	X

(continued)

89

INSURANCE COVERAGE FOR CONTRACEPTION *(continued)*

State	Private Insurance		State Employees		
	Coverage Required	Coverage Not Required	Coverage Required	Coverage Not Required	Coverage Available[1]
Indiana		X	X		X
Iowa	X		X		X
Kansas		X	X[7]		X
Kentucky	X[2]		X		X
Louisiana		X		X	X
Maine	X		X		X[10]
Maryland	X			X	X
Massachusetts		X[6]	X		X
Michigan		X[6]	X[7]		X
Minnesota	X[8]		X		X
Mississippi		X	X		X
Missouri		X	X		X
Montana		X[6]		X	
Nebraska		X		X	X
Nevada	X		X		X
New Hampshire	X		X		X
New Jersey	X[2,6]		X		X
New Mexico		X[5,6]		X	X
New York		X	X		X
North Carolina	X		X		X
North Dakota		X[6]		X	
Ohio		X[5,6]	X		X
Oklahoma	X[7]		X		X
Oregon		X	X		X
Pennsylvania		X	X		X
Rhode Island	X		X		X[10]
South Carolina		X		X	X
South Dakota		X	X		X
Tennessee		X	X		X
Texas	X[5,6]		X		X
Utah		X	X		X
Vermont	X		X		X
Virginia		X[4]	X		X
Washington		X[9]	X		X
West Virginia		X[6]	X		X
Wisconsin		X	X		X
Wyoming		X[6]		X	
Total	20	31	35	16	45

[1] An (x) in this category means that some type of insurance coverage for contraception is available in this state.

[2] These states require certain insurers in the small employer and/or individual markets to offer plans that provide coverage for contraception.

3 A statute requires insurers that cover prescription drugs to provide coverage for oral contraceptives.

4 This statute requires insurers to offer coverage for contraception as an employer option, but does not mandate coverage.

5 Statutes or regulations require HMOs to cover voluntary family planning services when medically necessary.

6 Statutes or regulations require HMOs to cover voluntary family planning services, but either this term is not defined or the regulation is not interpreted to require coverage for contraception.

7 A regulation requires HMOs to cover voluntary family planning services, interpreted to include some kind of contraception.

8 A statute requires HMOs to provide coverage for prescription drugs, interpreted to include coverage for contraception.

9 As of December 15, 2000, a rule was pending that would require insurers that cover prescription drugs to provide equitable coverage for contraception.

10 In these states, coverage pursuant to the new contraceptive coverage laws must be available on the date state employees' health plans are issued or renewed.

CHAPTER 3

CHRONOLOGY

1670s

■ Dutch scientist Antonie van Leeuwenhoek first views sperm under a microscope.

1790

■ The first modern gestation and delivery of a child conceived through artificial insemination is recorded.

1821

■ Connecticut enacts the first U.S. statute against abortion.

1841

■ Abortion has been made a crime in 10 of the 26 states as a result of routine revisions of legal codes throughout the United States.

1857

■ Horatio R. Storer, a Harvard-trained doctor specializing in obstetrics and gynecology, begins a national drive within the newly formed American Medical Association (AMA) to criminalize all induced abortions.

1866

■ Storer publishes *Why Not: A Book for Every Woman*, to convince women that, contrary to tradition, fetal life begins far earlier than "quickening" (the moment when the woman can feel the fetus moving).

Chronology

1867

■ Storer makes the same argument for a male audience in *Is It I?: A Book for Every Man*.

1868

■ Feminist activist and suffragist Elizabeth Cady Stanton refers to abortion as "the degradation of woman" in the first volume of *Revolution*, the suffragist journal; later that year her colleague, Matilda Gage, writes: "[T]his crime of 'child murder,' 'abortion,' 'infanticide,' lies at the door of the male sex."

1869

■ Pope Pius IX declares that all abortion is murder—the first time in its history that the Roman Catholic Church has taken such a position. Previously, Catholic tradition did not consider to be sinful abortions that took place before "quickening," when the pregnant woman first feels the fetus move, around the fourth or fifth month of pregnancy.

1870–71

■ "The Evil of the Age," a series of articles in the *New York Times*, focuses on abortionists, whom it portrays as profiteers exploiting innocent and vulnerable women. In describing the body of a woman who dies from a failed abortion, the *Times* refers to her as "a new victim of man's lust, and the life-destroying arts of those abortionists, whose practices have lately been exposed in the TIMES."

1873

■ Congress passes the Comstock Law, which explicitly defines as obscene all contraceptive devices and all information about contraception, making it a crime to send such devices or information through the U.S. mail. The Comstock Law also applies to any kind of sex education and any kind of noneuphemistic sexual information, such as the naming of genitalia (and to many other kinds of writing and images, including literary works and images deemed "obscene"). Anthony Comstock, head of the New York Society for the Suppression of Vice, is appointed a special agent to carry out the act. The law enables him to prosecute people who sell contraceptive devices as well as abortionists.

Reproductive Rights and Technology

1878

- Comstock arrests the country's richest and best-known provider of abortions, Madame Restell of New York City. Restell, expecting to be convicted, kills herself 24 hours before her trial.

1880

- As a result of the campaign by Storer and the AMA, some 40 antiabortion statutes have been passed. U.S. abortions are now considered criminal regardless of the point in the pregnancy at which they are induced. Whereas prosecution had formerly focused on abortionists, now it includes women receiving abortions as well.

1884

- Dr. William Pancoast, a Philadelphia medical school professor, is approached for help by a wealthy couple trying to have a child. Pancoast anesthetizes the wife, seeks the help of the best-looking medical student in his class, and injects the unconscious woman with semen from the first known U.S. sperm donor, unbeknownst to either the woman or her husband. Later, when the child comes to resemble the donor, Pancoast tells the husband the truth. The husband asks only that his wife never be informed.

1910

- The Eugenics Record Office is established in Cold Spring Harbor, New York, with the purpose of training field workers to gather family histories of people around the country. Their ultimate goal is to encourage the breeding of "good" families and to discourage the breeding of "bad" families to improve the genetic makeup of the United States. By 1924, data has been recorded on some three-quarters of a million cards, and the office routinely gets inquiries about whether proposed marriages would be genetically appropriate.

1914

- Birth control pioneer and socialist Margaret Sanger establishes *The Woman Rebel*, a feminist monthly magazine advocating birth control. As a result, Sanger is indicted for inciting violence and promoting obscenity.

1916

- Margaret Sanger opens the first U.S. birth control clinic with the goal of making contraceptive devices and family planning information available to poor women, which leads to her being jailed for one month.

Chronology

1921

- Margaret Sanger founds the American Birth Control League, which will later become the Planned Parenthood Federation.

1927

- The Supreme Court case of *Buck v. Bell* authorizes the sterilization of Carrie Buck on the grounds that she is feebleminded. Justice Oliver Wendell Holmes writes: "It is better for all the world if, instead of waiting to execute degenerate offspring for crime, or to let them starve for their imbecility, society can prevent those who are manifestly unfit from continuing their kind. ... Three generations of imbeciles is enough."

1929

- The ejaculate of U.S. men averages 90 million sperm per cubic centimeter.

1931

- Some 30 states have passed laws to sterilize people considered either to be "feebleminded" or to have "criminal tendencies."

1937

- "Conception in a Watch Glass," an editorial in the prestigious *New England Journal of Medicine*, proposes the notion of in vitro fertilization.

1938

- The first survival of sperm after freezing, known as cryopreservation, is recorded.

1942

- The American Birth Control League, which had been founded by Margaret Sanger in 1921, becomes Planned Parenthood Federation, the name under which it is known today. Planned Parenthood remains one of the most active organizations fighting for reproductive rights and providing reproductive health services to U.S. women.
- The Supreme Court rules in *Skinner v. Oklahoma* that a 1935 law allowing for the forced sterilization of certain kinds of criminals is unconstitutional. However, *Buck v. Bell* remains in force, so that the involuntary sterilization of the "feebleminded" is still allowed under the Constitution.

1953

■ The first successful human pregnancy from frozen sperm is recorded.

1954

■ In one of the first recorded U.S. legal cases involving artifical insemination (AI), an Illinois court rules that inseminating a married woman with the sperm from a man to whom she is not married constitutes adultery, even if her husband has consented.

1959–60

■ Two federal courts find that D.H. Lawrence's novel *Lady Chatterley's Lover* cannot be banned as obscene. Although the Comstock laws still provide the basis for obscenity trials and the banning of child pornography, this marks the beginning of the end for laws against sex education and birth control materials being sent in the mails.

1960

■ The U.S. Food and Drug Administration approves the birth-control pill, ushering in what some have called the Sexual Revolution. For the first time in human history, women of childbearing age can be heterosexually active and yet be almost completely certain of not getting pregnant.

1962

■ The American Law Institute publishes a proposed Model Penal Code, in which it recommends legalizing abortions in cases that would "gravely impair the physical or mental health of the mother"; when the child would be born "with grave physical or mental defects"; or "if the pregnancy resulted from rape or incest." These suggestions are far more liberal than the abortion laws in most U.S. states at the time.

■ The Sherri Finkbine case draws national attention to laws concerning abortion. Finkbine, a middle-class mother of four and host of the TV show *Romper Room*, takes the tranquilizer thalidomide while pregnant with her fifth child. When she reads that thalidomide is expected to produce severe birth defects, she arranges with her doctor for an abortion. At the time, Arizona law allows abortion only to save the woman's life. Out of concern for other pregnant women, Finkbine tells the Arizona *Republic* about thalidomide, asking that her name be withheld. When the story hits the front page on the morning that Finkbine's abortion is scheduled, the hospital cancels the abortion for fear of prosecution. Finkbine's doctor requests a court order for the operation; the judge dismisses the case and recommends the abortion. When the hospital continues to refuse, the Finkbines go to Sweden and have the abortion there. The fetus does indeed prove to be severely deformed.

As a result of the Finkbine case, President John F. Kennedy announces that the FDA will increase its regulation of potentially harmful medications and asks U.S. citizens to destroy any thalidomide tablets they may have. Kennedy also awards the country's highest civilian honor, the medal for Distinguished Federal Civilian Service, to Frances Oldham Kelsey, the FDA researcher who stood up to enormous corporate pressure and refused to approve thalidomide (a German drug) for manufacture in the United States.

The Vatican denounces the Finkbine abortion as murder.

1964

- An outbreak of German measles results in more than 20,000 congenitally deformed babies. (German measles, or rubella, can cause birth defects if the woman contracts it during pregnancy, particularly during the first trimester.) Doctors who perform abortions on pregnant women with rubella face the loss of their licenses.

1965

- Doctors, social workers, and theologians form the Association for the Study of Abortion in order to compile and circulate data on abortion, hoping to gain public support for revising the abortion laws.
- *June 7:* The Supreme Court decision *Griswold v. Connecticut* strikes down Connecticut laws that made it illegal for married couples to use contraception. The basis for the Court's decision is its recognition of the right to privacy, a legal premise that will be central to later reproductive rights decisions, including *Eisenstadt v. Baird* (1972) and *Roe v. Wade* (1973).

1967

- President Lyndon Baines Johnson approves an annual budget of more than $20 million for contraceptive programs, signaling a new public acceptance of "family planning."
- In a striking reversal of its initial position, the American Medical Association comes out in favor of legalizing abortion.

1968

- Although "first-wave feminists" like Elizabeth Cady Stanton saw abortion as something that men imposed upon women, "second-wave feminism" sees abortion as part of a woman's right to be sexual and to control her own body. After an initial period of uncertainty, the National Organization for Women (NOW) comes out in favor of making abortion legal.

- The National Association for the Repeal of Abortion Laws is founded.
- The Catholic Church outlaws oral contraceptives and all other "artificial" methods of birth control in the encyclical *Humanae Vitae*, written by Pope Paul VI.

1969

- The American Civil Liberties Union (ACLU) comes out in favor of legalizing abortion, beginning a history of pro-choice activism that continues to this day. It is joined by Planned Parenthood and the World Population Organization.
- Robert Edwards, the pioneering embryologist who will one day help create the first "test-tube" baby, publishes an article in *Nature* about artificially fertilizing human eggs.
- *January:* New York NOW founds New Yorkers for Abortion Law Repeal, which cites radical feminist principles as a basis for supporting the legalization of abortion. They are joined by the radical feminist group Redstockings. Both groups hold speak-outs and demonstrations, invade legislative hearings, and lobby against abortion reform campaigns that include medical restrictions on abortion. The feminist groups argue that abortion is not a medical decision but rather reflects a woman's right to have control over her body and her sexuality.
- *February:* The first National Conference on Abortion Laws is held in Chicago.
- *August 26:* Dramatic demonstrations to repeal antiabortion legislation are held in U.S. cities nationwide.

1970

- Alaska, Hawaii, and New York repeal their laws outlawing abortion.

1971

- Two new antiabortion groups are formed: Pro-lifers for Survival, an antinuclear group, and Feminists for Life.
- Congress deletes the portions of the Comstock Law that apply to contraception and abortion.
- Some 70 abortion-related criminal and civil cases are pending. The Supreme Court agrees to hear *Roe v. Wade* and *Doe v. Bolton*, which will become landmark cases when the decisions are rendered in January 1973.

Chronology

1972

- Since 1967, 14 states have passed laws to allow therapeutic abortions: Arkansas, California, Colorado, Delaware, Florida, Georgia, Kansas, Maryland, Mississippi, North Carolina, New Mexico, Oregon, South Carolina, and Virginia. (A therapeutic abortion is one deemed necessary to preserve the woman's life or health.)
- Vanderbilt University Professor Dr. Pierre Soupart becomes the first U.S. scientist to prove he can fertilize a human egg in vitro.
- In *Eisenstadt v. Baird* the Supreme Court rules that a Massachusetts law allowing the sale or distribution of contraceptives only to married persons is unconstitutional. The court finds that the right of privacy established in *Griswold v. Connecticut* (1965) extends to all individuals and thus protects the right of unmarried persons to obtain contraceptives.
- Native American mother Norma Jean Serena sues a number of hospitals in the Armstrong County, Pennsylvania, for damages relating to her sterilization in 1970, after the birth of her third child. Serena, who had been on welfare at the time of the birth, claims that she could not recall signing a consent form for the procedure. The case will not be settled until 1979.

1973

- Quebec resident Claude Vorilhon takes the name Rael and founds a group known as the Raelians. According to their gospel, the *Elohim*, or angels, of the Bible were actually aliens who had cloned human beings and whose gospel included the injunction, "Thou shalt clone."
- *January 22:* The Supreme Court hands down the decisions in *Roe v. Wade* and *Doe v. Bolton*, landmark decisions making abortion widely available to U.S. women. In *Roe*, a 7–2 majority finds that a woman's right to privacy includes the right to have unregulated abortions in the first trimester; the state is allowed to regulate abortions to protect women's health beginning in the second trimester, and to protect "the potential life of the fetus" in the third trimester. In *Doe*, other aspects of a Georgia law criminalizing abortion were considered, as the principles of *Roe* were reaffirmed.
- The National Association for the Repeal of Abortion Laws becomes the National Abortion Rights Action League (NARAL).
- *June:* In response to *Roe v. Wade*, the National Right to Life Committee is formed. This marks the beginning of national anti-abortion activism, which will come to be known as the "right to life" or "pro-life" movement.
- *September 12:* Floridians Doris and John Del Zio become the first U.S. couple to attempt in vitro fertilization (IVF), when their New York City

infertility specialist, Dr. William Sweeney, surgically removes an egg from Doris and has it fertilized by John. The fertilized egg is stored in an incubator by Sweeney's colleague, Dr. Landrum Shettles of Columbia Presbyterian Hospital. Shettles's supervisor, Dr. Raymond Vande Wiele, chair of Columbia's Department of Obstetrics and Gynecology, is furious with Shettles for participating in a risky procedure and interrupts the incubation process. As Doris's fallopian tubes were badly damaged, Sweeney did not believe he could surgically extract a second egg from them. When Doris learns that the IVF procedure has been interrupted, she falls into a profound depression.

1974

- Doris and John Del Zio file suit against Dr. Raymond Vande Wiele, Columbia Presbyterian Medical Center, and Columbia University, claiming that by interrupting the IVF procedure conducted by Drs. Sweeney and Shettles, Vande Wiele had destroyed Doris's one chance to be a mother.
- Dr. Pierre Soupart applies for funding from the National Institutes of Health (NIH) for a three-year $375,000 study to determine the safety of in vitro fertilization.
- *July:* Studies show that in this month alone, 48 sterilizations of Native American women have been performed and several hundred have been conducted in the previous two years, part of what Native American activists charge is an ongoing pattern of excessive and often coerced sterilizations.

1975

- *Spring:* Dr. Pierre Soupart is informed by NIH that he will receive the funds for which he had applied, but he must wait for the approval of the Ethics Advisory Board, which has not yet been appointed.
- The Supreme Court hands down *Bigelow v. Virginia*, voting 7–2 to strike down a Virginia statute that bans the advertisement of abortion services.
- The Supreme Court hands down *Connecticut v. Menillo*, unanimously upholding the way a Connecticut statute prohibiting the performance of abortion was used to prosecute a nonphysician. The Court points out that *Roe* allowed regulation of abortion to protect a woman's safety. The Connecticut statute, the Court finds, provides the minimum standard of safety on which *Roe* was predicated.
- The rate of sterilization for U.S. women has increased by 350% since 1970. Some activists charge that this is because of Indian Health Service and welfare department efforts to encourage or even coerce Indian women, other women of color, and women on welfare to be sterilized.

Chronology

1976

- *July 1:* The Supreme Court hands down *Planned Parenthood of Central Missouri v. Danforth*, finding unconstitutional a Missouri law that allows a woman's husband or parents to have the final say in a contested abortion.
- *September:* Attorney Noel Keane, who calls himself the "father of surrogate motherhood," claims to have arranged the first surrogate-mother contract when an infertile woman and her husband come to him for help. Keane will later arrange the contract between the Sterns and Mary Beth Whitehead in the infamous "Baby M" case.
- The Supreme Court hands down *Bellotti v. Baird (I)*, ruling unanimously that a federal district court should have abstained from deciding upon the constitutionality of a Massachusetts statute requiring parental consent for a minor's abortion. The Court held that before reaching the federal level, the statute ought to have been interpreted by the state court. As part of its decision, the Court notes that there are some circumstances in which a state may indeed require a minor to obtain a parent's consent before obtaining an abortion.

1977

- Congress passes the Hyde Amendment, named for Illinois representative Henry Hyde, attached to appropriations funding for what was then the Department of Health, Education and Welfare (now the Department of Health and Human Services). The amendment bans federal Medicaid funds from being used to pay for abortions, except those necessary to save the woman's life.
- In *Carey v. Population Services International,* the Supreme Court strikes down a New York law with three provisions: 1) a ban on the sale of nonprescription contraceptives by anyone other than a licensed pharmacist; 2) the sale or distribution of contraceptives to minors under 16; 3) the display and advertising of contraceptives. The Court finds that the New York statute violates adults' and minors' right to privacy and violates contraceptive vendors' right to free "commercial" speech.
- *June 20:* The Supreme Court hands down *Beal v. Doe*, in which it rules that a Pennsylvania decision to deny Medicaid funding for elective abortions (abortions not deemed medically necessary to save the woman's life) is indeed constitutional. In the Court's view, Medicaid plans are required to cover only "necessary" medical treatment, whereas elective abortions are considered "unnecessary (though perhaps desirable)." Moreover, the Court finds, "The State has a strong interest in encouraging normal childbirth that exists throughout the course of a woman's pregnancy" and it is permissible to further such an interest by refusing to subsidize non-

101

therapeutic abortions. Finally, the Court points out that when Congress passed the bill authorizing Medicaid funding, nontherapeutic abortions were illegal in most states, suggesting that the funding program was never intended to fund abortions.

- *June 20:* Again, in *Maher v. Roe*, the Court upholds a Connecticut state refusal to use Medicaid funding for elective abortions, finding that a state need not fund a woman's exercise of her right to abortion even though it pays for the cost of her childbirth.
- *June 20:* In *Poelker v. Doe*, the Supreme Court upholds a St. Louis municipal policy of refusing all publicly financed hospital services for elective abortions. According to this ruling, while abortion remains a woman's legal right, the State is not obligated to provide funds to help make this right accessible.

1978

- Researchers report a 126 percent increase in the number of abortions performed on the Navajo reservation since 1972. The rate of abortions per 1,000 deliveries has increased from 34 to 77.
- The NIH's Ethics Advisory Board begins its deliberation of Dr. Pierre Soupart's 1974 proposal to study the safety of IVF.
- *July 17:* The Del Zio suit goes to trial. The court awards John Del Zio $3 in damages for his lost sperm and gives Doris Del Zio $50,000 for her mental anguish.
- *July 25:* Louise Brown, the first "test-tube baby," is born. She is the child of English parents, Lesley and John Brown, and the IVF procedure was performed by pioneering embryologist Robert Edwards. The pregnancy had generated so much publicity that while the pregnant Lesley resided at the hospital, the medical facility was mobbed by reporters, including journalists disguised as boilermakers, plumbers, and window cleaners. Someone—believed to be a reporter—calls in a bomb scare to the maternity wing, hoping to get a glimpse of Brown as the building is evacuated.
- In response to Louise Brown's birth, right-to-life advocates persuade Illinois lawmakers that any doctors who fertilize a human egg in vitro have custody of the embryo and are thereby subject to Illinois' 1877 child abuse law.
- In what may be the earliest recorded example of harvesting a dead man's sperm, Dr. Cappy Rothman retrieves semen from a deceased unmarried 19-year-old, whose parents want to continue the family's lineage.

1979

- Norma Jean Serena's case, begun in 1973, is finally settled. Serena had charged several doctors and a male social worker with violating her civil rights by taking part in her sterilization. She claimed that she had never given consent to the procedure. The attending physician argues that he had explained the procedure to her and that she understood. The jury agrees with the doctor.

- *January 9:* In *Colautti v. Franklin*, the Supreme Court rules that a Pennsylvania law is both "void for vagueness" and unconstitutional. The law required a doctor intending to perform an abortion to determine that a fetus is not viable. Under the law, if a doctor found a fetus to be viable, he or she was required to exercise the same degree of care in performing the abortion that would have been exercised if the fetus were intended to be born alive. The Court found that this law was unacceptably vague, because the meanings of "viable" and "may be viable" were unclear. ("Viability" is the medical term used to refer to a fetus's ability to survive outside the womb.) Decisions on viability must be left to the good-faith judgment of the doctor, said the Court, not codified into law. Moreover, the law was unconstitutional in that it imposed a criminal liability on doctors, regardless of their intent to violate the law. In other words, if doctors acted in good faith to perform a legal abortion on what they believed to be a nonviable fetus, they might be charged with criminal liability despite their intentions to do no harm.

- *July 2:* The Supreme Court hands down *Bellotti v. Baird (II)*, in which it finds unconstitutional a Massachusetts law requiring 1) that a minor must attempt to obtain written consent from both parents before approaching a court for permission to get an abortion; 2) that the judge may deny the petition if he or she believes that an abortion is against the minor's best interests. Instead, says the Court, all minors must be able to approach a judge for approval of an abortion without notifying their parents and that the proceedings must be confidential. If the minor is mature, she must be allowed to have an abortion, whether or not the judge sees that procedure as in her best interests. If the minor is immature, the judge can determine whether an abortion is in her best interests—but if it is, the abortion must be confidential if the minor wishes.

- The ejaculate of U.S. men averages 60 million sperm per cubic centimeter, down from 90 million sperm/cc in 1929. Fertility specialists believe that environmental toxins may be responsible for the decline in male fertility.

- The first IVF is performed on baboons.

- Robert Klark Graham founds "Repository for Germinal Choice," a well-publicized sperm bank. Graham wants to limit sperm donors to Nobel Prize–winning male scientists and restrict female clients to those belonging to Mensa, an organization for people with high I.Q.s. Graham later relaxes his regulations to some extent, but his endeavor gains notoriety as an example of modern eugenics.

1980

- The first international meeting on IVF is held in Kiel, Federal Republic of Germany.
- Mary Ann Smedes, a 36-year-old unmarried woman, sues Wayne State University's infertility clinic on the grounds that its restriction of artificial insemination to married couples constitutes discrimination. Smedes is represented by the American Civil Liberties Union (ACLU), which charges that the clinic's policy violates her constitutionally guaranteed reproductive freedom and her right to equal treatment under the law. The case is never tried; rather it is settled when the university agrees to drop its marriage requirement and to consider Smedes for artificial insemination. However, Smedes does not proceed with insemination because of the vast number of threatening letters she has received from people who oppose the notion of single motherhood, and because clinic doctors indicate that they would discourage her on the grounds of age.
- *June 30:* The Supreme Court hands down *Harris v. McRae*, in which the Court finds the Hyde Amendment to be constitutional. The suit had challenged the amendment, which bans federal Medicaid funds from being used to pay for abortions except those necessary to save the woman's life. The Court finds that the government has no obligation to fund abortions, even if it chooses to pay for the cost of childbirth.
- *June 30:* The Supreme Court rules in *Williams v. Zbaraz* that Illinois's version of the Hyde Amendment is constitutional. Thus the state of Illinois—and by implication, other states—may ban state Medicaid funds to pay for elective abortions, even if they use Medicaid funds to pay the costs of childbirth.

1981

- *March 23:* In *H. L. v. Matheson*, the Supreme Court upholds a Utah law requiring a doctor to notify a parent of an "unemancipated minor" (a minor still under the parents' care) before an abortion. The Court pointed out that the minor seeking the abortion had made no claim that she was mature enough to give informed consent. Nor did she claim that she had problems with her parents that would make notifying them inappropriate. In the case of this minor, then, the law was valid. Justices Potter Stewart and Lewis Powell wrote a concurring opinion in which they emphasized that mature minors and those whose best interests required parents not to be involved would be entitled to a confidential abortion.

- *June 10:* Dr. Pierre Soupart dies without ever having been funded for his research into the safety of IVF.
- The first U.S. child of IVF is born, Elizabeth Carr. The IVF procedure was performed at the clinic of Howard Jones and Georgeanna Seeger.

1982

- The Sperm Bank of California is founded to make sperm donations available to unmarried heterosexual and lesbian women. Most sperm banks will provide sperm only to married, heterosexual couples.
- *April:* The first child of Robert Klark Graham's "Repository for Germinal Choice," is born. Victoria Kowalski's biological parents were among the high-intelligence men and women to whom Graham limited his services.

1983

- The first IVF is performed on chimpanzees.
- In *Bolger v. Youngs Drug Products Corporation,* the Supreme Court strikes down a federal law that had made it a crime to send unsolicited contraceptive advertisements through the U.S. mail. The Court finds that this law violates the First Amendment's protection of "commercial speech," and interferes with parents' access to information that might help them discuss birth control with their children. The fact that some people might be offended by the material, the Court rules, is not a valid reason for prohibiting the communication of truthful, nonobscene material.
- *June 15:* In *City of Akron v. Akron Center for Reproductive Health,* the Court strikes down as unconstitutional an Akron, Ohio, ordinance requiring that 1) a woman wait 24 hours between consenting to an abortion and actually receiving one; 2) all abortions after the first trimester be performed in full-service hospitals; 3) minors under the age of 15 have parental or judicial consent for an abortion; 4) the attending doctor personally give a woman information relevant to her informed consent; 5) specific information be given to a woman before an abortion, including details of fetal anatomy; a list of the risks and consequences of the procedure, some of which were false or hypothetical; and a statement that "the unborn child is a human life from the moment of conception"; 6) fetal re-

mains be "humanely" disposed of. The Court strikes down each provision on the following grounds: 1) The 24-hour waiting period did not serve the state's interest in protecting the woman's health nor in ensuring her informed consent; 2) Requiring hospitalization interfered with a woman's access to abortion without protecting her health, as certain abortions may safely be performed outside of full-service hospitals; 3) The minors' consent requirement did not guarantee an adequate judicial alternative (that is, there was no adequate provision for a judge to step in if parents were unavailable or if it was inappropriate to approach them); 4) Counseling by a doctor made abortions more expensive and such counseling was not really necessary to secure informed consent; 5) Providing doctors with particular scripts interfered with an individual doctor's judgment; moreover, such scripts were not neutral information but were in fact a means of persuading women not to exercise their legal right to have abortions; 6) Requiring "humane" disposal of a fetus was too vague a requirement to be legal. This ruling will be overturned in the 1992 decision, *Planned Parenthood of Southeastern Pennsylvania v. Casey.*

- *June 15:* In *Planned Parenthood of Kansas City, Missouri v. Ashcroft*, the Supreme Court ruled on a Missouri law requiring that 1) all post-first-trimester abortions be performed in hospitals; 2) two doctors be present at every abortion of a viable fetus; 3) a pathologist's report be obtained for each abortion; 4) minors under 18 have either parental or judicial consent for their abortions. The court found that 1) the hospitalization requirement added to the cost of an abortion without making it any safer, so it was struck down; 2) the requirement that two doctors be present at late abortions served the State's interest in protecting the potential fetal life that had been mentioned in *Roe v. Wade*, and so was constitutional; 3) the pathology report imposed only a small financial burden on the woman and protected her health, and so was constitutional; 4) the parental consent requirement included a "judicial bypass" provision and so was constitutional.
- *June 15:* In *Simopoulos v. Virginia*, the Supreme Court upholds the criminal conviction of a doctor who had been charged with violating a Virginia law requiring all post-first-trimester abortions to be performed in hospitals. The Court finds that Virginia law allows freestanding clinics to be licensed as "hospitals," and that Dr. Simopoulos could have avoided prosecution simply by licensing his clinic.
- A proposed constitutional amendment asserting that the right to an abortion is not secured by the Constitution is rejected by the Senate with a vote that falls 18 ballots short of the two-thirds majority required. The combination of the Supreme Court rulings and the Senate vote is considered a major setback for the pro-life movement and an endorsement of the "pro-choice status quo."

106

Chronology

1984

- The first-ever birth from an egg donation is reported in Australia.
- Lawrence Suscy, venture capitalist, enters into a partnership with physicist and cattle breeder Richard Seed, who has tried to adapt successful cattle-breeding techniques for use on human beings: A fertile woman is inseminated with a man's sperm and an embryo begins to develop. After a few days, the embryo is "flushed" from the fertile woman and implanted into an infertile woman (ideally, the sperm donor's wife). Suscy tells *Fortune* magazine that the new company, Fertility and Genetics Research, wants to develop a nationwide chain of fertility clinics. They plan to recruit hospitals to give them long-term, low-interest loans of $1 million in exchange for part ownership in a clinic. As the treatments will cost $4,000–$7,000, and as Suscy anticipates 30,000 to 50,000 candidates for treatment, he expects his venture to be highly profitable. "Volume is nothing, margin is everything," Suscy tells *Fortune*.
- *March 28:* Dr. Richard Marrs achieves the first U.S. birth of a frozen embryo, Zoe Leyland.
- Robert Klark Graham's former colleague, Paul Smith, opens his own "genius sperm bank," Heredity Choice.
- Pro-life physician Dr. Bernard Nathanson narrates *The Silent Scream*, a powerful video that purports to record an actual abortion on ultrasound. *The Silent Scream* is widely distributed, endorsed by President Ronald Reagan, and sent to every member of Congress. It is still used by pro-life groups today.

1985

- There are now 169 IVF clinics in the United States—although about half of them cannot claim a single successful live birth.
- Historian and lawyer Paul Lombardo conducts research on Carrie Buck, the allegedly feebleminded woman whose sterilization was authorized in the 1927 Supreme Court case, *Buck v. Bell.* Lombardo discovers that Buck was not feebleminded at all; in fact, both she and her daughter had done well in school. Rather, she was considered to be "immoral" for having a child out of wedlock—even though the child was the result of a rape by the nephew of the foster parents with whom she lived, and who were the ones who had her committed.

1986

- The first known birth from frozen eggs takes place under the care of an Australian doctor.

- Fertility and Genetics Research, the company of venture capitalist Lawrence Suscy and cattle-breeder Richard Seed, goes public on NAS-DAQ as BABY. Although at first the company raises $8 million, it goes on to lose money.
- The Supreme Court votes 5–4 in *Thornburgh v. American College of Obstetricians and Gynecologists* to strike down a Pennsylvania statute regulating abortions. At issue are five provisions: 1) doctors are supposed to give their parents specific information about abortion, including state-produced printed materials describing the fetus; 2) doctors performing abortions on viable fetuses must use the method most likely to result in fetal survival unless it would cause "significantly" greater risk to a woman's life or health; 3) a second doctor must be present at abortions of viable fetuses; 4) detailed reports on abortions must be filed and be available to the public for inspection and copying, to include the identification of the attending physician and information about the woman receiving the abortion; 5) either one parent's consent or a court order is required for a minor to obtain an abortion. The court strikes down the first four provisions and sends the issue of parental consent to the lower court, in light of newly enacted state court rules.

1987

- ***March:*** Fertility and Genetics Research announces that due to serious financial difficulties, it will not start the embryo transfer center it had planned.
- Dr. John Buster, a UCLA infertility specialist, patents the embryo transfer procedure he had worked on at Fertility and Genetics Research. The American Fertility Society's Ethics Committee condemns the patenting of a medical procedure as unethical. Buster's success in obtaining a patent starts a trend of other fertility specialists and geneticists patenting both procedures and portions of human genetic material.
- German doctors are successful at producing frozen-egg pregnancies.

1988

- The first U.S. child from a donated egg is born.
- The "Baby M" case is decided. New Jersey couple William and Betsy Stern had asked Mary Beth Whitehead to serve as a surrogate mother—but after the birth, Whitehead refused to surrender custody of the child. When a New Jersey Court temporarily awarded custody to Mr. Stern (who was the child's biological father), Whitehead fled with the baby, her husband, and her other two children. The court fi-

nally decides to award permanent custody to Mr. Stern, with White-head retaining parental rights and permission to make supervised visits. Mrs. Stern, who has no biological relationship to the child, is allowed no legal relationship, either.

■ A new pro-life group is formed, Operation Rescue, which will become known for its militant actions to frustrate the operations of abortion clinics.

1989

■ *York v. Jones* is decided. Risa York and her husband, Steven, had enrolled in Howard Jones's Virginia clinic and undergone in vitro fertilization, which resulted in the creation of several embryos. After four unsuccessful attempts to implant an embryo in Risa, the couple decided to have one of their embryos frozen for later use. When the Yorks moved to Los Angeles, they decided to continue fertility treatment there but were not allowed to remove the embryo from the Virginia clinic. A court order is finally needed before the Yorks recover the embryo in 1989 and take it with them to California.

■ *April 9:* Between 300,000 and 600,000 women and men march on Washington in the March for Women's Equality/Women's Lives, the largest march on Washington since the Vietnam War, partly spurred by women's fears of how the Supreme Court will rule in the upcoming case *Webster v. Casey.*

■ *April 26:* The Supreme Court hears oral arguments in *Webster v. Reproductive Health Services.*

■ *July 3:* The Supreme Court hands down *Webster v. Reproductive Health Services,* upholding a Missouri statute that finds that life begins at conception; bars the use of public funds for the purpose of counseling a woman to have an abortion that she doesn't need to save her life; bans abortions in public facilities; and requires doctors to perform tests on women pregnant for 20 weeks or more to find out whether fetuses are viable. This decision is seen as a turning point in Supreme Court rulings, as it opens the door for restrictive state regulations on abortion.

1990

■ Congress funds the Human Genome Project, a $3 billion undertaking whose goal is to map and analyze the 50,000 to 100,000 genes in the human cell. The project's first director is James Watson, codiscoverer of DNA.

■ *June 25:* The Supreme Court hands down *Hodgson v. Minnesota,* concerning a Minnesota law that requires both biological parents to be notified when a minor has an abortion, with a 48-hour waiting period between the notification and the abortion, and with no judicial bypass. The law made no exception for divorced or unmarried parents. However, a second section of the law did provide for a judicial bypass if a court ordered it. The law had been in effect for nearly five years by the time the case reached the Supreme Court. The Court found that the law's requirement of two-parent notification with no judicial bypass was unconstitutional; however the Court upheld the part of the law that would allow a court to require judicial bypass, as well as the 48-hour waiting period for minors.

- *June 25:* The Supreme Court rules on *Ohio v. Akron Center for Reproductive Health,* upholding an Ohio statute requiring a doctor performing an abortion on a minor to give notice to her parent or guardian 24 hours before the procedure. The law also provided for a judicial bypass, allowing a minor to get a court order rather than tell a parent. The Court rejected a challenge alleging that Ohio's complicated procedure for obtaining a judicial waiver was too burdensome for minors and therefore not constitutional. It upheld the requirement that the doctor must personally notify the parent.

1991

- Canada's Royal Commission on New Reproductive Technology discovers that lesbianism is considered grounds for refusal of treatment at 28 of 49 Canadian fertility programs.
- A 42-year-old South Dakota woman, Arlette Schweitzer, becomes pregnant with an egg donated by her daughter and sperm donated by her daughter's husband, thus becoming the "mother" of her own grandchild. Schweitzer undertakes the surrogate pregnancy because her own daughter was born without a uterus.
- *May 23:* The Supreme Court hands down *Rust v. Sullivan* and *State of New York v. Sullivan.* This case concerns a challenge to 1988 regulations of the U.S. Department of Health and Human Services (DHHS), banning staff at federally funded family planning clinics from counseling women about abortions, referring them to places where they might obtain abortions, or even from informing them that abortion is a legal option. The Court notes that the DHHS rule reverses 18 years of policies, but finds that the DHHS secretary has the right to change the policy based on a "shift in attitude toward the elimination of unborn children by abortion."
- In British Columbia, a woman wins the first lawsuit alleging HIV infection from donated semen. Another patient at the same clinic had received

the same semen and also tested HIV-positive, although she chose not to sue. The plaintiff is awarded $883,800 in damages, but the appeals court orders a new trial.

■ Representative Ron Wyden of Oregon introduces a bill that would have forced embryo laboratories within fertility clinics to be federally certified. However, the Bush administration vows to oppose federal intervention into matters that have been historically left to the states. Wyden writes a new version of his bill, requiring the Secretary of Health and Human Services to design a certification program for states to adopt and considers amending the bill to establish the American Fertility Society's guidelines on artificial insemination as "standards of care" for purposes of lawsuits regarding AI. Although the AFS supports federal certification of embryo laboratories, it opposes any federal regulation of clinical medicine. Wyden's bill does not become law.

1992

■ Through DNA testing, federal prosecutors prove that at least 15 and as many as 75 children born to the patients of fertility doctor Cecil Jacobson were created with the doctor's own sperm—unbeknownst to his patients.

■ A woman sues a New York sperm bank when she discovers that the sperm she has received is not that of her dying husband, but rather from a man of another race. The woman claims that her daughter has been subjected to racial prejudice as a result. The case is settled out of court for $400,000.

■ The Supreme Court refuses to hear *Davis v. Davis*, a case involving the once-married couple Mary Sue and Junior Davis, who had been receiving IVF that resulted in seven embryos, which were preserved for eventual implantation into Mary Sue's womb. The couple then began divorce proceedings. Mary Sue wanted to preserve the embryos, but Junior wanted them destroyed so that his wife could not implant them and sue him for child support. A lower court awarded Mary Sue custody of the embryos, but the Tennessee Supreme Court eventually ruled that Junior could not be forced to become a father against his will. When the Supreme Court refuses to hear the case, the embryos are returned to Junior, who destroys them.

■ *June 29:* In *Planned Parenthood of Southeastern Pennsylvania v. Casey*, the court votes 7–2 to explicitly overrule parts of its decisions in *Ohio v. Akron Center for Reproductive Health* (1990) and *Thornburgh v. American College of Obstetricians and Gynecologists* (1986). In this new case, the Court upholds parts of a Pennsylvania statute regulating abortions: 1) doctors are required to give their patients information about abortion, including pictures of fetuses at various stages of development; 2) women face a mandatory 24-hour delay following these lectures; 3) detailed reports on abortions must be filed and be available to the public for copying, to include the name and location of any state-funded facility that performs abortions; 4) a minor seeking an abortion must obtain the consent of one parent, with judicial bypass available. The justices strike down one provision of the Pennsylvania law, that which had required a married woman to obtain her husband's consent before receiving an abortion. While the Court affirms *Roe*, it also offers a radically new interpretation of that decision: Rather than viewing the decision to choose abortion as a fundamental right, the Court says instead that the State may impose no "undue burden" on this choice. The State may try to persuade a woman not to have an abortion, as long as it places no "undue obstacle" in her way while doing so. Four Justices vote to overturn *Roe* completely. The decision itself and the strong opposition to *Roe* is considered to signal a significant change in the Court's position on abortion and reproductive rights.

- *October 24:* Congress passes Public Law 102-493, the Fertility Clinic Rate and Certification Act of 1992, requiring fertility clinics to inform patients of their individual success rates (rather than nationwide average rates of success).
- *November:* Pro-choice president Bill Clinton is elected.

1993

- *January 13:* In *Bray v. Alexandria Women's Health Clinic*, the Supreme Court votes 5–4 to find that a federal civil rights law known as the "Ku Klux Klan" Act does not protect women from pro-life protestors who are obstructing their access to abortion clinics. The Court finds that pro-life blockades do not constitute sex-based discrimination for the purpose of this statute.
- The first U.S. birth from intracytoplasmic sperm injection (ICSI) is reported. ICSI is a procedure whereby a woman's eggs are harvested and injected in vitro with sperm; when an embryo results, it is implanted into the woman's uterus. The procedure makes it possible for men with low sperm counts to father children. Doctors begin offering ICSI more routinely, even though critics argue that fertile women are being put through a complicated medical procedure in response to their husband's infertility, not their own.
- President Clinton signs into law the National Institutes of Health Revitalization Act, which allows the federal government to fund research on IVF, with the goal of making it less expensive, more effective, and

112

safer. Despite the long-standing existence of IVF and related technologies, this is the first time the U.S. government has sponsored research in this area.
- *March:* Michael Griffin kills abortion provider Dr. David Gunn in front of his clinic in Pensacola, Florida.
- *August:* Oregon housewife Shelley Shannon shoots and wounds Dr. George Tiller, late-term abortion provider in Wichita, Kansas. Evidence seized after Shannon's arrest links her to arsons at clinics in four other states. Police find buried in Shannon's back yard correspondence between Shannon and two men imprisoned for abortion-related violence and a manual published by the militant pro-life group Army of God explaining how to attack abortion clinics.

1994

- The British make it illegal to harvest the eggs or ovaries of fetuses for use in fertility treatments.
- In *National Organization for Women v. Scheidler*, the Court rules on NOW's efforts to use the Racketeer Influenced and Corrupt Organizations (RICO) Act in a suit against pro-life organizations that unlawfully blockade or harass abortion clinics. NOW initiated the suit on behalf of abortion providers in Delaware and Wisconsin that had been blockaded by Operation Rescue, Pro-Life Action League, and other pro-life groups. RICO was established in 1970 as a tool against organized crime; it punishes "enterprises" that engage in a "pattern of racketeering." At issue is the question of whether pro-life blockades and clinic harassment constituted the kind of national conspiracy that RICO was intended to forbid. The Court unanimously finds that NOW could indeed use RICO as the basis for its suit, even though the nationwide conspiracy that NOW was alleging had no economic basis.
- In *Madsen v. Women's Health Center*, the Supreme Court votes 5–4 to uphold two major provisions of a Florida injunction: 1) a 36-foot buffer zone must be created outside the entrance to an abortion clinic; 2) pro-life protestors are prohibited from making noise that can be heard inside the clinic during the hours when surgical procedures are being performed. The Court overrules provisions of the law that would have created a 300-foot no-approach zone around the clinic; a ban on signs and images visible to people inside the clinic; and a 300-foot ban on picketing outside the residences of clinic employees. However, the court indicates that more narrow prohibitions on actual or veiled threats might indeed be constitutional.
- President Clinton vows that no federal funds will be awarded to research that uses human embryos.

- After Operation Rescue publicly disavows the killing of abortion providers, the American Coalition of Life Activists breaks away to form the ACLA, with the public goal of supporting the "justifiable homicide" of doctors who perform abortions.
- *May:* Congress passes the Freedom of Access to Clinic Entrances (FACE) Act, making it a federal crime to block access to clinics. Soon afterward, Janet Reno assigns federal marshals to defend clinics around the country.
- *July:* Guy Hudson is born. Guy's sisters, created in vitro at the same time as Guy, were born three years earlier, making Guy the first "time-warp triplet."
- *July 18:* At age 62, Rosanna della Corte delivers a 7-pound, 4-ounce son, thereby becoming the oldest woman ever to give birth. Della Corte was implanted with a donor egg fertilized by her husband's sperm.
- *August:* Paul Hill shoots Dr. John Britton and his escort, Lt. Col. James Barrett, in Pensacola, Florida. Hill had attended ACLA's conference.
- *December:* John Salvi III shoots and kills Shannon Lowey and Leanne Nichols, workers at two different abortion clinics in Brookline, Massachusetts.
- *December:* The Justice Department organizes a task force on pro-life violence, working in conjunction with a federal grand jury investigation.
- *December:* Since Bill Clinton's election in 1992, clinic-related violence has doubled. Since March 1993, five people have been killed in clinic violence.
- Moderates on each side of the abortion issue form Common Ground, in an attempt to find issues on which both sides can agree.

1995

- A national shortage of Pergonal, a widely used fertility medication that induces ovulation, leads the FDA to allow foreign imports of this drug.

1996

- The British Human Fertilisation and Embryology Act goes into effect, providing that frozen embryos may not be stored for longer than five years. The law is amended in May 1996 to extend the maximum storage time with the consent of both parents. British clinics are unable to locate the parents of many frozen embryos but are unwilling to destroy them— even as they are running short of money and storage space to preserve the embryos. The Vatican calls the destruction of the embryos "prenatal massacre." More than 3,300 English embryos are eventually destroyed.
- Arceli Keh becomes the oldest woman to give birth, at age 63, after lying about her age to fertility specialists.
- Dr. Ricardo Asch, a California fertility specialist, flees the country after being sued by Loretta and Basilio Jorge. The Jorges have learned that

114

Loretta's eggs and perhaps Basilio's sperm may have been used to impregnate another woman, while Loretta remained unable to conceive a child after 16 years of trying and $30,000 for two IVF procedures. Some 40 former patients joined the Jorges in their suit against Asch, while the Jorges sought partial custody for the child that resulted from Loretta's egg.

- *January:* The federal grand jury, convened in 1994, concludes that there is no evidence for a national conspiracy against abortion clinics. Smaller, regional investigations continue.
- *Spring:* Common Ground, a group dedicated to bringing together both sides of the abortion debate, holds its first national conference.

1997

- *January 1:* Section 367 of the California penal code goes into effect, making it illegal to steal eggs or embryos. The law was passed in response to the 1996 scandal involving Dr. Ricardo Asch.
- U.S. doctors are writing 1.3 million fertility drug prescriptions each year, for a total of almost $230 million.
- In *Schenck v. Pro-Choice Network of Western New York*, the Supreme Court votes 8–1 to strike down a New York injunction that creates a 15-foot "floating" buffer zone around any person or vechicle seeking to enter or leave a clinic. However, the Court limits this holding to the facts of this particular case, noting that it did not address the question of whether a "zone of separation" might ever be necessary. The Court votes 6–3 to uphold a provision creating a 15-foot "fixed" buffer zone outside of clinic doorways, driveways, and parking lot entrances. The Court also upholds a "cease and desist" provision that allowed a pregnant woman trying to enter the clinic to ask protestors to withdraw, in which case, the protestors had to retreat 15 feet from the person they had approached and remain outside of the buffer zone.
- In *Mazurek v. Armstrong*, the Supreme Court reverses a lower court ruling that would have permitted health-care providers to challenge a Montana law that bans supervised, licensed physician's assistants from performing abortions. The Court found that, in general, physician-only requirements are indeed constitutional.
- The cloning of Dolly the sheep just outside Edinburgh, Scotland, represents the first successful cloning of a large mammal. Dr. Ian Wilmut and his team perform the procedures that lead to Dolly's creation.
- In response to Dolly's cloning, Rael forms Ventures, a Bahama-based cloning operation. He also forms Clonaid, a group dedicated to cloning humans. Rael offers places on the waiting list for his operation in exchange for $200,000; within a short time, he has collected $2 million and hired scientists to begin research into human cloning. He also starts a project known as Insuraclone, which for $50,000 allows parents to store

cells from a living child so that they might clone a second child if the first one dies. Later he starts Clonapet, to allow people to clone their pets.

- The University of California at Irvine, where Dr. Ricardo Asch had practiced, settles with the Jorges for $650,000, part of an $18.4 million settlement given to 61 couples.
- *February 2:* After sixteen years of trying to conceive, Loretta Jorge gives birth to a baby boy conceived without fertility treatments.
- An Italian surrogate mother is found to have carried embryos from two different couples. DNA testing is needed to sort out the parentage of the children.
- In an unprecedented move, California shuts down Heredity Choice, the "genius sperm bank" founded by Robert Klark Graham's former colleague, Paul Smith. The state finds that the clinic has no running water and lacks basic hygiene. The state has also heard charges that dog semen samples were commingled with human ones, as dogs were also bred at the clinic. Heredity Choice challenges the state action.
- The first U.S. woman gives birth to a baby conceived from a frozen egg.
- *November:* Bobbi McCaughey becomes the first known mother of septuplets, resulting from the fertility procedures she had undergone.
- *November:* An article in *Fertility & Sterility* reports on South Korean researchers who found that eggs that had been frozen, then thawed, had more chromosomal abnormalities than non-frozen eggs. The researchers claim that freezing itself hurts DNA.

1998

- *January 29:* An abortion clinic in Birmingham, Alabama, is bombed, killing an off-duty police officer and seriously wounding a nurse.
- *March:* A New Jersey court makes its final custody ruling in the case of "JayCee B," a child conceived via an egg donated by one woman, fertilized by sperm from an anonymous donor, and implanted in a third woman—who was carrying the child to term for John and Luanne Buzzanca, an infertile couple living in New Jersey. When John had filed for divorce in 1995, a month before the baby was born, he refused to pay child support, on the grounds that the child was not genetically his, even though he had signed the surrogacy contract. The surrogate, Pamela Snell, then sued for custody, arguing that she had agreed to carry and deliver the child on the understanding that it would be born into a stable, two-parent family. The egg donor also stepped forward, claiming that the egg had been used without her permission; followed by the sperm donor and his wife, who claimed that the sperm had been used without his consent. Neither donor sued for custody, and eventually, Snell withdrew her

claim. The court finally awards custody to Luanne Buzzanca and requires John Buzzanca to pay child support.

- *May:* In what may be the first instance of this procedure, a woman uses sperm collected after a man's death to get pregnant.

1999

- The first "IVF grandchild" is born. Natalie Brown, the younger sister of Louise Brown and herself an IVF baby, gives birth to her own daughter, Casey, establishing that children resulting from IVF procedures are capable of producing their own children. Natalie conceived Casey without fertility treatments.
- A Louisiana Senate judiciary committee passes a law giving an embryo the right to sue from the point of conception. The bill was inspired by a case in which a couple sought compensation for the pain and suffering of their stillborn child. The Louisiana Supreme Court ruled that while parents could sue for these damages, the stillborn child could not. The bill is part of a growing trends to recognize "fetal rights" as separate from the rights of the woman carrying the fetus.
- *September 30:* The House of Representatives overwhelmingly passes H.R. 2436 in a 254–172 vote. The so-called Unborn Victims of Violence Act would have become the first federal law to elevate all stages of prenatal development—starting with the embryo—to the legal standing of a person, whose rights are separate from and equal to those of the woman carrying the embryo or fetus. The law is written as an anticrime bill, and creates a separate criminal offense if a person causes death or injury to a person "who is carried in the womb." The bill would provide the maximum available punishment, even if the person who causes the fetal death did not know that the woman was pregnant.
- *October 21:* The Senate affirms its support for *Roe v. Wade* in a narrow 51–47 vote expressing the "Sense of the Senate" that *Roe* is "an appropriate decision and secures an important constitutional right."

2000

- *June:* The American Medical Association (AMA) supports community access to a full range of reproductive services after hospital consolidations. At issue is a series of mergers across the nation in which Catholic facilities join with secular ones—and institutions stop offering abortions as a result. The AMA initially considers a strong statement holding that any hospital providing services to pregnant women and receiving taxpayer money—including Medicaid and Medicare—must provide a full range of reproductive services. However, after receiving criticism from Roman Catholic leaders, the AMA approves a dramatically weaker amended resolution that stops short of saying that Catholic hospitals should perform all reproductive health procedures, including abortions, vasectomies, and tubal ligations (sterilization of women), all of which are prohibited by the Catholic Church. The AMA also votes to oppose gag clauses that prevent doctors from discussing abortions and other options with their patients.

- In *Hill v. Colorado*, the Supreme Court considers a challenge to a Colorado statute that establishes an eight-foot "bubble zone" around anyone within 100 feet of a health-care facility. The law, aimed against pro-life protestors, would keep them from approaching without consent closer than eight feet to anyone within 100 feet of a clinic entrance, with the purpose of leafleting, showing a sign, or engaging in protest, education, or counseling. The statute is being challenged on the grounds that it violates the First Amendment. The Court finds that the statute is indeed constitutional, because it allows for a reasonable restriction that is not based on the content of a person's speech and that offers ample alternative means of communication. For example, a protestor may stand still and allow a person to approach him or her.

- The Rebecca Corneau case in Massachusetts attracts national attention. Corneau, a member of a small religious community, asserts that seeking medical care violates her religious beliefs. She and her community are suspected of neglect in the death of Corneau's last baby as well as some other children from her community. When Corneau is taken into protective custody to force her to get what social service groups consider appropriate medical care, pro-choice feminists get involved in defending her. These feminists assert that they disagree with Corneau's choice but they are concerned with the precedent of jailing a woman because of her conduct during pregnancy.

- *June 28:* In *Stenberg v. Carhart*, the Supreme Court votes 5–4 to strike down a Nebraska ban on so-called "partial-birth" abortion. "Partial-birth" abortion is a colloquial phrase that Nebraska argued referred only to the so-called dilation and extraction (D&X) procedure. However, the Court finds that the law is so broadly written that it would also ban "a much broader category of procedures," including the "dilation and evacuation (D&E)" procedure, the most commonly used method in second-trimester abortions. Moreover, the Nebraska law contains no provision for exceptions that might be needed to protect a woman's health. For these reasons, the court finds that it creates an undue burden on a woman's right to abortion.

- *August 29:* Adam Nash is born. The child was conceived specifically in order to be a blood donor to his six-year-old sister Molly, who suffers from Fanconi anemia, a preleukemia condition. Adam was conceived through IVF so that the doctors could conduct pre-implantation genetic diagnosis, a procedure whereby embryos are monitored for genetic defects before being implanted into the woman's womb. Adam was conceived from an embryo determined to be free of Fanconi anemia, so he was known to be a genetically healthy match for Molly. A transfusion from Adam's umbilical cord into Molly's veins was begun soon after Adam was born, a treatment with an 85%–90% success rate. Adam's birth provokes a firestorm of controversy about the ethics of creating one life for the purposes of supporting another.

- *September 28:* The Food and Drug Administration (FDA) approves mifepristone, or RU-486, popularly known as "the abortion pill."

2001

- *January 22:* President George W. Bush bans federal aid to international organizations that perform or "actively promote" abortion as a family planning method. Groups that mention abortion as an option will no longer qualify for U.S. funds.
- *January 28:* Leaders on both sides of the abortion debate have been meeting secretly in the Boston area for nearly six years, in the wake of the John Salvi shootings; they publicly disclose the results of these conciliatory talks and call for new mutual understanding.
- *February 2:* The Senate confirms Missouri senator John Ashcroft as U.S. Attorney General after a bitter five-week struggle ending in a 58–42 vote in Ashcroft's favor. Ashcroft is known for his long history of militant pro-life stands, but he says during confirmation hearings that he will uphold *Roe v. Wade* because it is the law of the land.
- *March:* Congressional critics of President Bush's January 22nd action have been seeking a way to release federal funds for pro-choice family planning abroad. President Bush issues a new order imposing abortion restrictions on foreign aid, in an effort to implement a different legal strategy that will frustrate the efforts of his opponents.
- *June 6:* The pro-choice group, the Center for Reproductive Law and Policy, brings suit in Federal District Court in Manhattan, arguing that the rights of free speech and political association are violated by President Bush's January 22nd decision to deny federal funds to foreign family planning and to health organizations that perform or advocate abortions.
- *June 12:* A federal judge in Seattle rules that a family-owned drugstore chain discriminated against women when it failed to include prescription contraceptions in its employee health plan. The Seattle case is the result of a class-action lawsuit filed in July 2000 by Jennifer Erickson, a pharmacist at Bartell Drug Company. Erickson claimed that the company's health insurance plan violated the Pregnancy Discrimination Act, since the plan provided for all the health needs of male employees, even as female employees had to pay for their own contraception.

Reproductive Rights and Technology

- *July:* The Jones Institute for Reproductive Medicine in Norfolk, Virginia, announces that it is creating human embryos for the sole purpose of medical research, fueling the ongoing controversy over this issue within the Bush adminstration and the Republican Party. Some anti-abortion Republicans, like Senator Orrin Hatch of Utah, support stem cell research, while Represenatitive Chris Smith, Republican of New Jersey, opposes both abortion and stem cell research. Health and Human Services Secretary Tommy Thompson, while an adamant foe of abortion, was a strong supporter of stem cell research at the University of Wisconsin during his tenure as governor of that state.
- *July 3:* A state appeals court in California upholds a state law requiring employers to cover contraceptives in their prescription drug plans. The law had been challenged by Catholic Charities, who had argued that the law infringed on the religious freedom of employers.
- *July 6:* The Food and Drug Administration (FDA) announces that a controversial type of fertility treatment will now come under its regulation. While the FDA had always maintained that it had the power to regulate fertility treatments, this is the first time it has chosen to exercise that power. The regulations concern a technique in which fluids from a young, fertile woman's egg are injected into the egg of an older, infertile woman's egg before the older woman's egg is fertilized by her partner's sperm, leading to the unprecedented mixing of three kinds of genetic material rather than two. The procedure is pioneered by Barnabas Medical Center in Livingston, New Jersey, but some half-dozen clinics are known to offer the procedure. The FDA requires that fertility doctors fill out an investigational new drug application (IND) if they want to mix male and female genetic material in any way other than the uniting of sperm and egg. The IND is the form that pharmaceutical companies must complete when the want to test a new drug on human subjects.
- *July 6:* The Bush administration seeks to define a fetus as an "unborn child" so that low-income pregnant women who do not qualify for Medicaid can qualify for a federal insurance program limited to children. The news comes to light when the draft of a letter by Dennis Smith, director of the Center for Medicaid and State Operations, is leaked to the press. Smith oversees the State Children's Health Insurance Program (SCHIP), which provides federal funds to states in order to cover medical insurance for families that do not qualify for Medicaid but cannot afford their own insurance. Reproductive rights groups are outraged by the move, which they see as a "back door" move to create legal rights for fetuses, including their own right to health care. Abortion opponents support the idea.
- *July 10:* The Wisconsin Supreme Court upholds a probation order barring a man convicted for failing to pay child support from having more

120

children unless he shows that he can support all of his offspring. Wisconsin resident David Oaks, father of nine children by four women, owes $25,000 in child support. As a result of the ruling, Oaks faces up to eight years in prison if he violates the order.

- *July 11:* Inspired by the June 12 ruling mandating Bartell Drug Company to include prescription contraceptives in its employees health-care plan, the Washington state chapter of the National Abortion and Reproductive Rights Action League (NARAL) and the American Civil Liberties Union (ACLU) bring suit against the Seattle-based Regence BlueShield insurance company, in an effort to require it to cover prescription contraceptives.

- *July 14:* The *British Medical Journal* reports on a new DNA test that might allow doctors to detect Down syndrome in embryos during IVF before the embryo is implanted in the womb. Currently, Down syndrome is most often tested for about 16 weeks into the pregnancy, using a sample of amniotic fluid from the pregnant woman's womb. The new test would be conducted during preimplantation genetic diagnosis (PGD), after the embryo has been created but before it has been implanted.

- *August:* At a National Academy of Sciences symposium, three doctors announce their intention to clone humans. One is Dr. Brigitte Boissellier, a chemist who is also a member of the Raelians, a religious sect committed to cloning. The second is Dr. Panayiotis Michael Zavos, who runs several medical laboratories in Kentucky. The third is Dr. Antinori Severino, the controversial fertility specialist. Their announcement comes a week after the U.S. House of Representatives votes to ban cloning, even for medical research.

- *August 14:* The New Jersey Supreme Court upholds a woman's right to decide whether frozen embryos produced by her and her ex-husband through IVF during their marriage can be implanted in another woman. The court rules that the seven embryos produced by the couple cannot be used to create a child without the woman's consent. The court does allow the father to maintain the frozen embryos indefinitely at a New Jersey in vitro clinic. Anti-abortion groups, which have long maintained that embryos represent life, are disappointed in the ruling, while reproductive rights groups supported the ruling.

- *September:* The Massachusetts high court, the Supreme Judicial Court, hears a case about whether children conceived posthumously from their late father's frozen sperm are eligible for Social Security benefits. The Social Security Administration has ruled that because the twins were born after their father's death, an 1836 state law requires them to be considered illegitimate. The children's mother, Lauren Woodward, has conducted a series of legal battles to have her late husband recognized as the children's legitimate father. Observers note that the current state of medical science was clearly not anticipated by the framers of the 1836 law.

Reproductive Rights and Technology

- **September 5:** The U.S. 9th Circuit Court of Appeals rules that male prisoners have a constitutional right to procreate by means of artificial insemination. The initial suit was brought by William Reno Gerber, a 41-year-old third-time convict serving an 111-year sentence for negligently discharging a firearm, making terrorist threats, and possessing a handgun as an ex-felon. Gerber wanted to send a semen sample to a medical center in Chicago, to be used to impregnate his 46-year-old wife. The ruling is supported by civil liberties groups, which cited a 1978 Supreme Court ruling allowing prisoners to marry. It is opposed by some conservatives, who raise eugenics arguments, among the Sacramento lawyer Ron Zumbrun, founder of the Pacific Legal Foundation, who asks, "If you are having lifetime criminals furthering their genes, is that in the best interests of society?"

- **September 6:** Massachusetts's Supreme Judicial Court (SJC) hears the case of Marla and Steven Culliton, the genetic parents of twins that were carried during pregnancy and borne by a surrogate who has no interest in raising them. Despite the surrogate's wish that the Cullitons act as the parents of their genetic child, the Cullitons were not given the parental rights they sought before their children were born. Although a 1998 SJC case allows genetic parents to have their names placed on birth certificates, a probate judge finds that adoption law prevents birth mothers from legally giving up their parental rights before birth. The SJC hears the Cullitons' case when the prematurely born children are seven weeks old.

- **September 15:** Dr. Robert G. Edwards, responsible for the first test-tube-baby birth in 1978, receives an award from the Albert and Mary Lasker Foundation for his pioneering work in fertility medicine. Edwards also pioneered stem-cell research and research into preimplantation genetic diagnosis, a technique that allows embryos to be screened for some genetic diseases before they are implanted in IVF procedures. He has also helped open the field of stem-cell research.

- **September 28:** The *New York Times* reports on a letter in which fertility specialist John Robertson, acting head of the American Society for Reproductive Medicine's ethics committee, expresses his support for a procedure by which prospective parents can screen embryos for sex. Embryos of an "unacceptable" sex can be discarded before they are ever implanted into the woman's womb. Robertson's statement draws outrage from other fertility specialists, although Dr. Norbert Gleicher, who had asked for Roberton's opinion, says that his own nine fertility centers readily offer the procedure. Another center offer a sperm-sorting technique that allows parents to extract the vast majority of male sperm, which it provides to couples who already have one child. Specialists distinguish, however, between sperm sorting and the destruction of an actual embryo.

CHAPTER 4

BIOGRAPHICAL LISTING

Dr. Severino Antinori, an Italian physician who has pioneered techniques for overcoming infertility. Antinori has helped some 70 postmenopausal women to become pregnant. He is responsible for the July 18, 1994, birth of a son to Rosanna della Corte, who at 62 years old was then the oldest known woman in the world to give birth (still older women gave birth in later years).

Ricardo Asch, the world-famous infertility specialist who pioneered the gamete intra-fallopian transfer (GIFT) technique, in which an egg and sperm are inserted into a woman's fallopian tube, so that fertilization can occur there instead of in vitro. This is one of the few reproductive techniques that has the approval of the Vatican, since it seems to resemble "natural" (unassisted) reproduction. Asch, a physician, had a clinic at the University of California at Irvine, which became the subject of a 1996 scandal when Asch was accused of using a drug on patients that had not been approved by the Food and Drug Administration (FDA). He was also accused of taking eggs and fertilized embryos from some patients and implanting them into other patients, without any of the parties' consent. One couple treated by Asch, Loretta and Basilio Jorge, sued for custody of the twins that they later discovered had been born using Loretta's eggs. Eventually, there were 84 lawsuits against Asch, his colleagues, and the university. In response, Asch fled to Mexico. As a result of the scandal, the California legislature passed a 1997 law making it a crime to use a woman's eggs or a couple's embryos without their consent. Asch now oversees an infertility clinic in Mexico and serves as international editor for the prestigious scientific journal *Human Reproduction.*

John Ashcroft, the Missouri senator and former attorney general of that state who became President George W. Bush's Attorney General in 2001; known for his strong objections to abortion. Because of his pro-life stance, Ashcroft's nomination provoked a controversy among feminist and pro-choice groups, among other constituencies. During his Senate hearings, Ashcroft made it clear that he opposed *Roe v. Wade* but said that he would accept it as settled law. He also stated that restricting abortion had been a hallmark of his career; that he opposes abortion even in cases of rape and incest; that he believes life begins at conception; and that he favors an amendment to the Constitution outlawing abortion. He also asserted that he would enforce laws against attacks on abortion clinics.

Baby M, Melissa Stern, the child who gave her name to the Baby M case, in which New Jersey couple William and Betsy Stern had asked Mary Beth Whitehead to serve as a surrogate mother, conceiving a child with William's sperm and carrying it to term. After the birth, Whitehead refused to surrender custody of the child, whom the Sterns had named Melissa. Because Whitehead had another name for her, the child became known in the news as Baby M. When a New Jersey Court temporarily awarded custody to William Stern, on the grounds that he was the child's biological father and would be a better parent than Whitehead, Whitehead fled with the baby, her husband, and her other two children. In 1988, the court finally decided to award permanent custody to William, with Whitehead retaining parental rights and permission to make supervised visits. Elizabeth Stern, who had no biological relationship to the child, was on that ground awarded no legal relationship.

Gary Bauer, president of the Family Research Council (FRC) and seeker of the Republican presidential nomination in 2000. During the 1980s, the FRC was one of the most influential Christian Right groups in Washington, and it provided major political and theoretical support for the pro-life movement. The Family Research Council was the research wing for James Dobson's group, Friends of the Family, best known for its opposition to gay rights but also an opponent of abortion, the distribution of condoms to teenagers, and other aspects of reproductive choice.

Harry Blackmun, the Associate Supreme Court Justice, appointed in 1970 by President Richard M. Nixon, known for writing the majority decision for the landmark 1973 *Roe v. Wade* decision, which overturned most existing state restrictions on abortion. Blackmun continued to be an outspoken advocate for abortion rights until he resigned from the Court in 1994. He died on March 4, 1999, at the age of 90.

Louise Brown, known as the world's first "test-tube baby"; actually the first child to be born successfully through in vitro fertilization (IVF). She is the child of Lesley and John Brown, and the procedure was performed by pioneering embryologist Robert Edwards. In response to Louise Brown's birth in July 1978, right-to-life advocates persuaded Illinois lawmakers that any doctors who fertilized a human egg in vitro had custody of the embryo and were thereby subject to Illinois's 1877 child abuse law.

Patrick "Pat" Buchanan, the 2000 Reform Party presidential candidate, formerly a Republican Party leader who had served in the administrations of Presidents Nixon, Ford, and Reagan, and who had sought the Republican presidential nomination in 1992 and 1996; a major political voice in the right-to-life movement. Buchanan claimed responsibility for returning the 1996 Republican platform to the pro-life policies of the Reagan years, and said that frustration with the Republican candidates who insisted on taking pro-choice positions despite the party platform had led him to leave the party and run on the Reform ticket.

Carrie Buck, the subject of the 1927 Supreme Court case, *Buck v. Bell,* in which Buck's sterilization was authorized on the grounds that she was feebleminded. Buck, an unwed mother, lived with a family for whom she worked as a servant. They institutionalized her and sought to have her sterilized. In a famous decision, Justice Oliver Wendell Holmes defended the practice of forced sterilization of the "unfit": "It is better for all the world if, instead of waiting to execute degenerate offspring for crime, or to let them starve for their imbecility, society can prevent those who are manifestly unfit from continuing their kind. . . . Three generations of imbeciles is enough." In 1985, research by historian Paul Lombardo revealed that neither Buck nor her child was feebleminded; rather, Buck's "feeblemindedness" had been inferred from her being an unwed mother, making her by definition immoral. In fact, Buck's pregnancy was the result of having been raped by the nephew of the family that had had her committed.

John and Luanne Buzzanca, the couple involved in a landmark 1988 custody case involving an egg donor, a sperm donor, a surrogate mother, and two adoptive parents (the Buzzancas). Their child, "JayCeeB," was born in 1995, a month after John filed for divorce. John had refused to pay child support, on the grounds that the child was not genetically his, even though he had signed the surrogacy contract. The surrogate, Pamela Snell, then sued for custody, arguing that she had agreed to carry the child on the understanding that it would be born into a stable, two-parent family. A New Jersey court finally awarded custody to Luanne Buzzanca and required John Buzzanca to pay child support.

Dr. M. C. Chiang, a collaborator with Dr. Gregory Goodwin Pincus, the inventor of the first effective oral contraceptive. Pincus and Chiang developed the pill with financing from Katherine Dexter McCormick, who also supported the clinical trials conducted by Dr. John Rock. The birth-control pill was approved by the FDA in 1960.

Anthony Comstock, head of the New York Society for the Suppression of Vice, and the force behind the Comstock Law, which Congress passed in 1873, explicitly defining as obscene all contraceptive devices and all information about contraception, and making it a crime to send such devices or information through the U.S. mail. The Comstock Law also applied to any kind of sex education, such as the naming of genitalia, and to the mailing of pornography, erotic literature, and any other literature or images that censors considered "obscene."Comstock was appointed a special agent to carry out the act. The law enabled him to prosecute abortionists and people who sold contraceptive devices.

Rebecca Corneau, a member of a small religious community in Massachusetts who in 2000 asserted that seeking medical care would violate her religious beliefs. She and her community are suspected of neglect in the death of Corneau's last baby as well as some other children from her community. When Corneau was taken into protective custody to force her to get what social service groups consider appropriate medical care, pro-choice feminists became involved in defending her. These feminists assert that they disagree with Corneau's choice but they are concerned with the precedent of jailing a woman because of her conduct during pregnancy.

Rosanna della Corte, at the time the oldest known woman to have given birth; her 7-pound, 4-ounce son was born on July 18, 1984, when della Corte was 62. Della Corte had been implanted with a donor egg fertilized in vitro with her husband's sperm, in a procedure conducted by the Italian fertility specialist Dr. Severino Antinori. As a result, Italy passed regulations resticiting the types of women who could receive certain kinds of fertility assistance, limiting the access of older women, lesbians, and single women.

Mary Ware Dennett, a feminist activist whose pamphlet, "The Sex Side of Life: An Explanation for Young People," led to her conviction under the Comstock Law. Dennett's conviction was reversed on appeal in a famous 1930 opinion by Judge Augustus Hand, *U.S. v. Dennett*, which was the first in a series of cases that gradually eroded the power of the Comstock Law. A colleague and then a rival of activist Margaret Sanger, Dennett founded the National Birth Control League and later the Voluntary Parenthood League to lobby for the repeal of state and federal bans on birth-control devices and information. Dennett wanted reproductive choice decisions to rest entirely with the woman involved, whereas Sanger favored a "doctors only" approach in which authority to dispense contraceptive devices and information lay with the medical establishment.

Robert Edwards, a Cambridge embryologist and pioneer of in vitro fertilization, responsible for the 1978 birth of Louise Brown, the world's first "test-tube baby" (baby conceived through IVF). Ironically, Edwards's work with IVF had been funded by a Ford Foundation grant whose ultimate goal was to develop contraceptives.

Jerry Falwell, a minister and political leader who in the 1970s helped to galvanize the Christian Right into activism against abortion rights and on many other social issues. Falwell was the founder of the Moral Majority, which later became known as the Liberty Lobby, a powerful religion-based group formed to mobilize support for a number of issues, including the right-to-life movement. He and his organization continue to be a powerful voice against abortion rights and other reproductive rights issues, such as distribution of condoms to teenagers.

Ruth Bader Ginsburg, Associate Supreme Court Justice, considered one of the "pro-choice" justices; the second woman ever to be on the Supreme Court, Ginsburg was nominated to the Supreme Court in 1993 by President Bill Clinton, who had run on a pro-choice platform. Ginsburg's nomination was initially resisted by feminists and abortion rights activists because she had been critical of the Supreme Court's reasoning in *Roe v. Wade.* Ginsburg said that she would have favored a more gradual approach in which state abortion laws might be liberalized over time, in order to avoid a political backlash. At her confirmation hearings, however, Ginsburg said that the right to choose an abortion was "something central to a woman's life, to her dignity . . . And when government controls that decision for her, she's being treated as less than a full adult human being responsible for her own choices."

Roger Gosden, a pioneer fertility scientist who hopes to develop a new birth control pill that will also delay menopause. Called "the career pill," the method would store eggs for use at a later date, so that women who were no longer ovulating naturally would have stored eggs that they might use to get pregnant after the age of 50.

Robert Klark Graham, an optometrist and inventor who founded the Repository for Germinal Choice, where he collected the sperm of Nobel prize–winning scientists and later, other geniuses. Access to the sperm was limited to women who were members of Mensa, an international society of people whose IQ tests certify them as among the most intelligent 2% of the population.

Dr. David Gunn, the first physician murdered for providing abortions; killed on March 10, 1993, by Michael Griffin outside a Pensacola,

Florida, clinic. Gunn had begun work as an infertility specialist, but when he established a practice in the rural South, he was committed to providing the full range of gynecological services, including abortions, to the largely poor and rural women in his practice who had very little access to medical care.

Paul Hill, the fundamentalist preacher who on July 29, 1994, murdered abortion provider Dr. John Bayard Britton and Britton's volunteer escort, James Barrett, and wounded Britton's wife, June, as the three arrived at a clinic in Pensacola, Florida. Hill had been inspired by Michael Griffin's murder of Dr. David Gunn outside the same clinic a year earlier and had achieved national prominence by going on the "Donahue" television show to talk about militant responses to abortion. Hill's crime was considered a turning point in moving mainstream public opinion to condemn pro-life violence; it also inspired Attorney General Janet Reno to create a Justice Department task force to investigate a potential conspiracy behind the nationwide violence. No evidence of a conspiracy was ever found.

Henry Hyde, the Illinois congressman who sponsored the 1977 Hyde Amendment, denying Medicaid payments for abortion; also a promoter of legislation to make federal health insurance available to poor women. Hyde has been a national leader in the right-to-life movement.

Cecil Jacobson, a Virginia physician who specialized in infertility treatments, a pioneer in reproductive technologies, and a onetime professor at George Washington University; the man who introduced amniocentesis (a method of prenatal screening for chromosomal abnormalities) into the United States. He was the subject of a 1992 federal investigation charging that from 15 to 75 children born to his patients had been created with his own sperm. He was also accused of telling one couple that their children were being created with the husband's sperm, when he in fact used his own sperm. Moreover, he gave some female patients hormone injections that created symptoms mimicking pregnancy, in some cases leading them to believe for up to 23 weeks that they were in fact pregnant, supported by ultrasounds and Jacobson's claims that he could hear their babies' heartbeats. One woman was made to believe she was pregnant three separate times. Jacobson appealed his case to the Supreme Court but was finally sentenced to five years in federal prison beginning in February 1994 and ordered to pay $75,000 in fines and refund $39,205 in patients' fees. He was also sued for child support by six couples whose children had been created with his sperm.

Dr. Howard Jones, along with his wife, Dr. Georgeanna Seeger Jones, the pioneers of IVF in the United States; the mentor of Robert Edwards. The couple were both professors at Johns Hopkins School of Medicine; they later retired to the Eastern Virginia Medical School. They were responsible for the 1981 birth of the first IVF child in the United States, Elizabeth Carr.

Arceli Keh, a 63-year-old woman who gained notoriety when she gave birth in 1996 after lying about her age to fertility specialists. Keh's case set off a debate about how old parents should be and about the ethics of doctors either facilitating the pregnancies of older patients or refusing treatment based on their own judgments about parental fitness.

Dorothy Kenyon, a feminist lawyer and judge on the board of the American Civil Liberties Union (ACLU); a leader in the ACLU's Reproductive Rights Project and a pioneer in fighting for women's right to choose both contraception and abortion.

Victoria Kowalski, the first child born using the "genius sperm bank" of Robert Klark Graham. Kowalski was born in April 1982 to Joyce and Jack Kowalski. This birth set off a controversy when it was learned that Joyce had lost custody of two children, Donna and Eric, from a previous marriage because she and her new husband, Jack, had abused them in order to make them "smarter," including beating them with a belt or strap when they made mistakes on the extra homework the parents gave them, and making Donna wear a sign on her forehead that said "Dummy."

Harry Laughlin, the pioneering U.S. eugenicist who headed the Eugenics Record Office in Cold Spring Harbor, New York, when the office was founded in 1910. Laughlin was responsible for publishing a Model Eugenical Sterilization law in 1914, which became the model for the law passed by Virginia in 1924 under which Carrie Buck was sterilized, as authorized by the famous 1927 Supreme Court decision *Buck v. Bell.*

Zoe Leyland, the first child born after having been frozen at the embryo stage. Zoe had been frozen as an embryo in an Australian clinic for two months before being implanted in her mother's womb. The year after her birth on March 28, 1984, there were 289 frozen embryos in the United States; there are now more than 100,000, increasing at the rate of nearly 19,000 per year.

Paul Lombardo, the researcher who discovered the truth behind the Supreme Court case of *Buck v. Bell.* In 1927, Buck's forced sterilization had been authorized by the U.S. Supreme Court on the grounds that she was feebleminded. Lombardo discovered that both Buck and her child were of normal intelligence, but Buck had been institutionalized for having borne a child out of wedlock.

Richard Marrs, a fertility specialist working with IVF who in 1985 achieved the first birth from a frozen embryo in the United States.

Katharine Dexter McCormick, a philanthropist who contributed up to $180,000 per year for several years to help finance the development of the first oral contraceptive, which was finally approved by the FDA in 1960. McCormick was heir to the International Harvester fortune, one of the first women graduates of the Massachusetts Institute of Technology, and a passionate feminist.

Norma McCorvey, the woman who used the pseudonym "Roe" in the landmark 1973 Supreme Court case, *Roe v. Wade.* Although McCorvey made history by seeking an abortion in that case, she later claimed she had been "used" by the feminist movement and became active with right-to-life groups. In 1995, she proclaimed her conversion to Christianity and founded the "Roe No More" ministry. In 1998, she published (with Gary Thomas) *Won by Love,* an autobiographical account of her experiences as a pro-choice activist and abortion clinic worker. In that book, McCorvey describes her alienation by what she considered to be the snubs of upper-class feminists; she claims to have been won over by the warmth and caring of the Operation Rescue activists who picketed the clinic where she worked.

Kate Michelman, longtime head of the National Abortion Rights Action League (NARAL), one of the major activist groups fighting for reproductive choice.

Hermann Muller, the winner of the 1946 Nobel Prize for his work demonstrating that X rays cause genetic mutations; an advocate of a sperm bank that would select male and female parents based on genetic traits considered to be desirable. For a while, Muller was associated with Robert Klark Graham, who seemed to be developing the kind of sperm bank that Muller had envisioned. Muller severed his relationship with Graham, however, on the grounds that Graham was trying to develop only intelligent children, not altruistic ones. To the distress of Muller's widow, Graham nevertheless named his facility after Muller.

Adam Nash, the first baby conceived specifically in order to be a blood donor. Adam's six-year-old sister Molly, suffered from Fanconi anemia, a preleukemia condition. Adam was conceived through IVF so that the doctors could conduct preimplantation genetic diagnosis (PGD), a procedure whereby embryos are monitored for genetic defects before being implanted into the woman's womb. Adam was conceived from an embryo determined through PGD to be free of Fanconi anemia. His birth provoked a firestorm of controversy about the ethics of creating one life for the explicit purpose of supporting another.

Bernard Nathanson, pro-life activist, the narrator and creator of *The Silent Scream,* a powerful video that purported to record an actual abortion on ultrasound. In 1968, Nathanson was a cofounder of the National Association for the Repeal of Abortion Laws, which later became the National Abortion Rights Action League (NARAL); he was also the director of the then-largest abortion facility in the world, New York City's Center for Reproductive and Sexual Health. In 1973, he became director of obstetrics at a New York City hospital, where he set up a prenatal research unit. He credits this experience, and the technology of ultrasound, with awakening in him the scientific certainty that life begins at conception, leading to a long career as a national spokesperson for the right-to-life movement. Nathanson has also told the story of having performed an abortion on a woman pregnant with a child that he himself had fathered. In 1996, Nathanson converted to Catholicism. He is now is a member of the American Bioethics Advisory Commission, a group formed by the American Life League to ban human cloning. He is the author of an autobiography, *Hand Of God* (1996).

John T. Noonan, Jr., one of the most important philosophers of the pro-life movement, author of the book *A Private Choice: Abortion in America in the 1970s* (1979), which portrays abortion as an antiwoman policy implemented by upper-class men. Noonan also edited a major reference work called *The Morality of Abortion: Legal and Historical Perspectives* (1970). In 1985, he was appointed by President Ronald Reagan to the Ninth Circuit U.S. Court of Appeals.

Sandra Day O'Connor, Associate Supreme Court Justice, first woman on the Supreme Court, known for her moderate pro-choice position, despite her generally conservative views on other matters. In *Stenberg v. Carhart* (2000), she was part of the narrow 5–4 majority that struck down Nebraska's ban on "partial-birth" abortion; she also helped write the majority decision in *Planned Parenthood v. Casey* (1992), striking down Pennsylvania state laws restricting women's access to abortion, including a provision that a married woman's husband must be notified. However, in 1989, in *Webster v. Reproductive Health Services*, O'Connor voted with the majority to uphold a Missouri statute that limited access to abortion in a decision that is generally viewed as having opened the door to state restriction of abortion rights. O'Connor was appointed by President Ronald Reagan in 1981. She attended Stanford law school with Chief Justice William Rehnquist.

John Cavanaugh O'Keefe, known as "the father of the rescue movement," the militant form of pro-life protest that involved trying to "rescue" women and fetuses from abortions by stopping women on their way into abortion clinics, engaging in "sidewalk counseling" to convince women not to have abortions, blocking access to the clinics, and otherwise trying to prevent the ongoing functioning of the clinics. He is currently director of Pro-Life Century, a division of Pro-Life Action League, one of the two original militant pro-life groups (Operation Rescue was the other). He takes credit for having caused the closing of more than 400 abortion clinics. He is an active opponent of human cloning and has recently written on the relationship between abortion, racism, and eugenics.

David N. O'Steen, executive director of the National Right to Life Organization, the largest and most established right-to-life group in the United States.

Dr. William Pancoast, the first physician known to practice artificial insemination. In 1884, Pancoast, a Philadelphia medical school professor, was approached by a wealthy couple trying to have a child. He anesthetized the wife, sought the help of the best-looking medical student in his class, and injected the unconscious woman with semen from the first known U.S. sperm donor, unbeknownst to either the woman or her husband. Later, when the child came to resemble the donor, Pancoast told the husband the truth. The husband asked only that his wife never be informed.

Dr. Gregory Goodwin Pincus, known as the "father of the Pill," the scientist who with Dr. M. C. Chiang and with financing by Katherine Dexter McCormick, developed the first effective oral contraceptive. Pincus and Chiang were encouraged by Margaret Sanger. Pincus was a professor at Boston University while conducting his research.

Dr. Martin Quigley, a physician at the University of Texas Health Science Center in Houston, founder of the second IVF clinic in the United States. Quigley has been an outspoken critic of IVF, pointing out that it has not been sufficiently studied and may lead to birth defects.

William Rehnquist, an Associate Justice of the Supreme Court since 1972 (appointed by President Richard Nixon) and Chief Justice since 1986 (appointed by President Ronald Reagan); author of the leading dissenting opinion in *Roe v. Wade* (1973), in which he argued that the framers of the fourteenth Amendment had never intended "equal protection under the law" to extend to a woman's right to abortion. Rehnquist was long considered one of the most conservative justices on the Court, though the appointments of Antonin Scalia and Clarence Thomas have given him colleagues with whom he is closely allied. All three are strict constructionists who believe that their job is not to promote a vision of society but rather to interpret the Constitution narrowly, restricting the role of government as much as possible. Rehnquist has voted to limit abortion rights in virtually every Supreme Court case since *Roe*, often writing the leading decision for his side.

Dr. John Rock, an obstetrician/gynecologist, Harvard medical school professor, and devout Catholic who conducted the clinical trials of the first effective oral contraceptive, which the Food and Drug Administration eventually approved in 1960. "The Pill" was developed by Drs. Gregory Goodwin Pincus and M. C. Chiang, with financing from Katherine Dexter McCormick. Rock considered "the Pill" to be a natural contraceptive because of its reliance on hormones that were naturally found in women's bodies. The Roman Catholic Church had long looked with disfavor upon contraception and explicitly prohibited oral contraceptives along with all other "artificial" means of birth control in 1968.

Margaret Sanger, a feminist and socialist activist who pioneered the acceptance of birth control in the United States. In 1914, she founded *The Woman Rebel*, a feminist monthly magazine that promoted birth control, based on Sanger's work among poor and immigrant women on New York's Lower East Side. Launching the magazine led to Sanger's indictment for inciting violence and promoting obscenity. In 1916, she opened the first family planning clinic in the United States, in Brooklyn, New York, which eventually led to her being jailed for a month. In 1921, she founded the American Birth Control League, which eventually became the Planned Parenthood Federation, an organization that still exists today. Widely considered the "founding mother" of reproductive rights in the United States, she has also been criticized for her sometimes narrow views, dictatorial attitudes, and, eventually, condescension toward the poor. However, she is also credited with galvanizing a national movement that led to a dramatic reversal in U.S. attitudes toward contraception and reproductive rights.

Antonin Scalia, an Associate Justice of the Supreme Court, appointed by President Ronald Reagan in 1986, known for his strong opposition to abortion, to *Roe v. Wade,* and to the Supreme Court's role in reproductive rights cases. Scalia has frequently written that abortion is a matter that ought to be decided by the people through their elected representatives, not by the Supreme Court; thus, if state legislatures wish to pass laws limiting access to abortion or outlawing it altogether, the Court has no business interfering, particularly since abortion is not a right guaranteed by the Constitution. Scalia is known for his colorful, abrasive style, which has alienated even fellow conservative Chief Justice William Rehnquist, with whom Scalia often votes. His devotion to "originalism"—the belief that the text of the Constitution should hold the key to any legal decisions that the Court makes—has had a profound effect on both liberal and conservative justices, moving them to justify their decisions less in terms of practical results and more in terms of how they fulfill the intentions of constitutional language. Scalia is personally a devout Roman Catholic, who worships with his wife at a suburban Virginia church known for its opposition to reproductive choice; in the late 1990s, the church erected a monument to unborn children.

Joseph Scheidler, founder in 1980 of the Chicago based Pro-life Action League (PLAN), one of the new, more militant right-to-life groups that emerged in the 1980s. Unlike the older groups, which worked through lobbying and legislative efforts, PLAN and a similar group, Operation Rescue, relied on "direct action," civil disobedience, and various types of harassment of clinic patients, doctors, and staff. Scheidler is the author of *Closed: 99 Ways to Stop Abortion*, in which he argued for the "doctrine of necessity," supporting the use of violence as a means of preventing greater violence.

Dr. Joseph Schulman, a pioneer of preimplantation genetic testing (PGD), which involves removing one cell of an eight-cell embryo, freezing the remaining seven, and testing the first cell for genetic defects. In this way, patients may request that only those embryos free of genetic disease be implanted into the mother's womb. Schulman was one of the first researchers to see a human embryo through a microscope (in 1974) and was the first director of the Medical Genetics Program at the National Institutes of Health, where he served on the faculty from 1973 to 1983. In 1984, he founded one of the first privately owned, for-profit infertility clinics, the Genetics and IVF Institute, which performs hundreds of IVF procedures a year.

William B. Shockley, the Nobel Prize–winning physicist who has argued that intelligence, as measured by performance on an IQ test, is inherited, so that categories of people who score low on IQ tests are genetically inferior. Shockley's arguments have been used to assert that African Americans are genetically inferior. Shockley has proposed that the U.S. government offer incentive payments to "genetically inferior" couples to become sterilized, at a rate of $1,000 for each IQ point below the norm. He has been called a "modern eugenicist" by critics who disagree with his theories of intelligence.

Dr. Pierre Soupart, the first U.S. scientist to prove that he could fertilize a human egg in vitro; he did so in 1972. A professor at Vanderbilt University, Soupart applied for National Institutes of Health (NIH) funding in 1974 to study the safety of IVF. Although Soupart was technically awarded a grant, a series of bureaucratic and political obstacles delayed the award; when he died in 1981, he had still not received the promised funding.

William and Elizabeth Stern, the New Jersey couple who made the surrogate motherhood arrangements with Mary Beth Whitehead that resulted in the birth of Baby M. After the birth, Whitehead refused to surrender custody of the child, whom the Sterns had named Melissa. When a New Jersey Court temporarily awarded custody to William Stern (who was the child's biological father), Whitehead fled with the baby, her husband, and her other two children. In 1988, the court finally decided to award permanent custody to William Stern, with Whitehead retaining parental rights and permission to make supervised visits. Elizabeth Stern, who had no biological relationship to the child, was on that ground denied a legal relationship.

Horatio R. Storer, the Harvard-trained obstetrician/gynecologist who in 1857 began a national drive within the newly formed American Medical Association (AMA) to criminalize all induced abortions. In 1866 and 1867, respectively, Storer published *Why Not: A Book for Every Woman* and *Is It I?: A Book for Every Man* to convince readers that, contrary to legal tradition, fetal life begins far earlier than "quickening" (the moment when the woman can feel the fetus moving, and the previously accepted legal definition of life's beginning). By 1880, as a result of Storer's and the AMA's campaign, some 40 antiabortion statutes had been passed throughout the United States. Storer had succeeded in branding abortions as criminal regardless of when in the pregnancy they were induced.

Randall Terry, founder and longtime leader of Operation Rescue, one of the best-known and most influential militant pro-life organizations of the late 1980s and early 1990s; later an unsuccessful Republican congressional candidate in New York. Terry was known for pioneering such tactics as "sidewalk counseling," in which women approaching abortion clinics were surrounded by at least two Operation Rescue protestors trying to convince them not to have an abortion and perhaps showing them pictures of fetuses, handing them literature, or calling them names. He also encouraged other militant techniques, including various forms of civil disobedience. Part of a strict Christian sect, he was censured in 2000 by his own church for leaving his wife and behaving "improperly" with other women, a charge Terry denied (while admitting that he was having marital difficulties). Terry is currently focusing on opposing gay and lesbian marriage and on another antigay activities, as is Operation Rescue, which he no longer heads.

Clarence Thomas, Associate Justice of the Supreme Court, appointed in 1992 by President George Bush after a bitter confirmation hearing in which Anita Hill, who had worked under him at the Equal Employment Opportunity Commission (EEOC), testified that he had sexually harassed her; known for his deeply conservative views and pro-life position. Thomas has stated that he would overturn *Roe v. Wade* if he could and has voted with Chief Justice William Rehnquist and Justice Antonin Scalia on abortion cases, in which the three conservative justices consistently vote in favor of individual states' rights to limit access to abortion.

Tommy Thompson, former governor of Wisconsin, chosen as Secretary of Health and Human Services by President George W. Bush; a strong opponent of abortion.

Don Treshman, director of Rescue America, one of the most militant pro-life groups of the mid-1990s. Treshman's Houston-based group was sued in 1994 by the family of Dr. David Gunn, the abortion provider slain outside a clinic in Pensacola, Florida, on the grounds that Rescue America had helped incite the killer, Michael Griffin. While Treshman denied those charges, he did solicit donations for Griffin's family within two hours of Gunn's murder, calling Gunn's death "unfortunate" but adding, "the fact is that a number of mothers would have been put at risk today and over a dozen babies would have died at his hands." In 1995, Treshman moved his operation to Baltimore, Maryland, after a Texas jury ordered Rescue America and other pro-life protestors to pay $1 million to a Planned Parenthood chapter. The protestors were found guilty of conspiring to hinder business at several Houston clinics in 1992. Today, Treshman works as public relations director of Human Life International, another militant pro-life group. He has also worked with the American Coalition of Life Advocates (ACLA), a group founded by pro-life activists who were unwilling to denounce the murders of abortion providers.

Daniel Ware, activist in Rescue America, a militant Houston-based pro-life group; friend of Paul Hill, convicted for the murder of a doctor and his escort; arrested in Pensacola, Florida, in early 1994 with a carload of weapons and more than 400 rounds of high-velocity ammunition. Ware had vowed to "terminate" abortion providers who had gathered in Pensacola for a memorial service for Dr. David Gunn, assassinated last year by another Rescue America member, Michael Griffin. Ware was prosecuted for saying that he intended "to take out . . . child-killers in a Beirut-style massacre." He was found not guilty by a Florida jury.

James Watson, first director of Human Genome Project, a federally funded project dedicated to mapping the human gene; Watson had won the Nobel Prize for his role in discovering DNA.

Biographical Listing

Sarah Weddington, the Texas lawyer and feminist activist who brought suit in *Roe v. Wade*, a lawsuit that resulted in the landmark 1973 *Roe v. Wade* Supreme Court decision. Weddington has continued to work as an advocate for reproductive rights.

Nancy Wexler, a pioneer in identifying and testing for the gene that results in Huntington's chorea, a debilitating genetic disease that, unlike most such diseases, does not appear until late in adulthood, so that would-be parents cannot know whether or not they are carriers. The test Wexler helped develop means that couples can create embryos in vitro and screen them for Huntington's disease before implanting them, eliminating any embryos infected with Huntington's. Wexler's research and its use in preimplantation genetic diagnosis (PGD) has fueled the debate among geneticists, fertility specialists, and disability activists about the extent to which parents should actively prevent the birth of disabled or otherwise challenged children.

Mary Beth Whitehead, the surrogate mother who gained prominence in the Baby M case, in which New Jersey couple William and Elizabeth Stern arranged for Whitehead to conceive and carry a child created with Stern's sperm. After the birth of the child, whom the Sterns named Melissa, Whitehead refused to surrender custody. When a New Jersey Court temporarily awarded custody to William Stern, Whitehead fled with the baby, her husband, and her other two children. In 1988, the court finally decided to award permanent custody to William, with Whitehead retaining parental rights and permission to make supervised visits. Elizabeth Stern, who had no biological relationship to the child, was therefore awarded no legal relationship.

Jack Willke, with his wife, Barbara Willke, founder of the 10-million-member National Right to Life Committee (NRLC) in 1980, the largest and most established pro-life group, which Willke headed for 10 years. Willke, a physician, began his activist career in 1970 when he and his wife founded Right to Life of Greater Cincinnati. He pioneered the technique of using dramatic visuals—particularly images that came to be known as the "Willke slides," featuring appealing images of fetuses that resembled babies and grisly pictures of fetuses after abortion. One photograph of a garbage bag full of discarded fetuses was reprinted in thousands of books and flyers. The Willkes' *Abortion Handbook* was known as the Bible of the pro-life movement and sold more than 1.5 million copies in 10 languages. When Willke resigned from the NRLC presidency in 1991, he went on to head the Cincinnati-based International Right to Life Federation and Life Issues Institute, which produces pro-life literature and radio commentaries. Barbara Willke served for a while as executive director of Right to Life of Greater Cincinnati before retiring in 1999 at the age of 76.

Stephen and Risa York, the plaintiffs in *York v. Jones*, a 1989 court case involving a couple's right to remove an embryo they had created from one fertility clinic and take it to another. Risa Jones and her husband, Steven, had enrolled in Howard Jones's Virginia clinic and undergone in vitro fertilization, which resulted in the creation of several embryos. After four unsuccessful attempts to implant an embryo in Risa, the couple decided to have one of their embryos frozen for later use. When the Yorks moved to Los Angeles, they decided to continue fertility treatment there but were not allowed to remove the embryo from the Virginia clinic. A court order was finally needed before the Yorks could recover the embryo in 1989 and take it with them to California.

CHAPTER 5

GLOSSARY

abortifacient   A substance or medication that produces an abortion.

abortion   The termination of pregnancy before birth, with the resulting death of the fetus. A spontaneous abortion, also called a miscarriage, occurs when the pregnant woman has an accident or disorder that prevents her from carrying to term; or when the fetus has a disorder that prevents it from developing normally and results in its demise. An induced abortion is intentionally brought on, either for health reasons or because the pregnancy is unwanted. An induced abortion may also be called a therapeutic abortion. Induced abortions may be either elective (by choice, when the woman's life is not at risk) or emergency (when the woman's life is immediately at risk).

adoptive parent   Man or woman who has chosen to care for a child and obtained legal custody of him or her, although he or she did not contribute sperm or egg toward the child's creation. The gap between biological and legal or adoptive parents has become wider as couples are arranging for egg and sperm donation and surrogate motherhood.

alternative insemination (AI)   A means of insemination (fertilizing an egg) other than through sexual intercourse, such as by introducing sperm into the woman's body through a catheter or fertilizing an egg in vitro.

amicus brief   *Amicus* is short for *amicus curiae*, or "friend of the court." A brief is a legal argument submitted in writing. An *amicus* brief or *amicus curiae* brief is a brief submitted by someone not directly involved in a case who nevertheless has an interest in its outcome. For example, in a case involving an abortion provider and a state official, *amicus* briefs may be submitted by religious groups, pro-choice groups, pro-life groups, the U.S. government, and other interested parties.

amniocentesis   A prenatal test in which a woman's amniotic fluid is sampled and examined; used to determine whether a fetus has any chromosomal abnormalities, such as Down syndrome (a form of mental retardation), as well as to test for other conditions of the pregnant woman

139

or fetus. Women over the age of 35 are at increased risk of giving birth to children with Down syndrome because of the increased age of their eggs.

artificial insemination (AI)   See *alternative insemination.*

assisted reproductive technology (ART)   The techniques used to assist a couple in producing a child, including alternative insemination (AI), in vitro fertilization (IVF), ovulation-inducing medications, gamete intrafallopian transfer (GIFT), and a variety of other means of overcoming infertility.

barren   An old-fashioned term for infertility in women.

biological parents   The woman and man whose egg and sperm created a particular child; as opposed to adoptive parents, nonbiological parents who have obtained legal custody of a child. The gap between biological and legal or adoptive parents has become wider as couples are arranging for egg and sperm donation and surrogate motherhood.

birth control   Methods used to prevent conception and pregnancy, also known as contraception. Birth control—the prevention of a pregnancy—can be contrasted to abortion, the termination of a pregnancy.

catheter   A tube used to transfer fluid.

cervix   The narrow opening between a woman's vagina and her uterus. During birth or during an abortion, the woman's cervix is dilated, or opened, to allow passage of the child or fetus.

Christian Right   A term developed in the 1980s for groups that used religion as the basis for their political activity. One of the central issues for organizations on the Christian Right was abortion, which they saw as murder.

clone   A genetic duplicate; or the act of creating a genetic duplicate.

compelling interest   A legal term referring to reasons that the State might take action, especially action restricting something that is otherwise considered a legal right. For example, in *Roe v. Wade*, the Supreme Court ruled that women's right to an abortion was guaranteed under the Fourteenth Amendment, but that the State might have a compelling interest to protect women's health by regulating abortions after the second trimester and to protect the potential life of the fetus by regulating abortions after the third trimester. If abortions are indeed guaranteed under the Fourteenth Amendment, the State needs a compelling interest to regulate them; otherwise, it is infringing upon a woman's right.

conception   The process of an egg being fertilized by a sperm to create a potential life.

constitutional   Legal under the U.S. Constitution; permitted under the Constitution.

contraception   Something that prevents (goes "counter to") conception. See *birth control.*

controlled ovarian hyperstimulation (COH)   The stimulation of a woman's ovaries to produce eggs in far greater numbers than usual, achieved through fertility drugs.

cryopreservation   Preservation through freezing; a method used to preserve embryos that have been created through IVF.

D&C (dilation and curettage)   Formerly the most common form of abortion but less often used since the development of vacuum induction. In a D&C, the woman's cervix is dilated and then her uterus is curetted, or scraped with a curette, a surgical tool that resembles a spoon. The curettage removes the fetus from the woman's uterine wall and carries it out through the woman's dilated cervix.

D&E (dilation and evacuation)   The most common form of second-trimester abortion. In a D&E, the cervix is dilated; then suction and a large curette are used to remove matter from the uterus, along with a large forceps that is used to grasp and extract the fetus. After week 15, the fetus may need to be dismembered before it can be removed. After 20 weeks, the fetus may be injected with intrafetal potassium chloride or digoxin to cause fetal demise before the fetus is evacuated.

D&X (dilation and extraction)   A form of second-trimester abortion that is generally used later in the pregnancy. The woman's cervix is dilated, the fetus is drawn out partway through the vaginal canal, feet first, and suction is used to remove the brain and spinal fluid from the fetal skull. The skull is then collapsed so that the fetus can be completely removed from the uterus. In this case, the fetus may be dismembered as it is pulled through the cervix, so that it can be removed. This procedure has been inaccurately termed "partial-birth abortion."

donor   Giver; an egg donor provides an egg that another woman will carry to term; a sperm donor provides the sperm that will fertilize an egg.

ectopic pregnancy   A pregnancy in which the fertilized egg implants in the fallopian tube rather than in the uterus. Ectopic pregnancies endanger a woman's life and cannot be carried to term; if they are not detected in time, they may require an emergency abortion. Also called tubal pregnancy.

ejaculate   Semen or "come"; the liquid that a man produces when he reaches orgasm; also used as a verb, meaning "to release semen by coming to orgasm": When a man ejaculates, semen shoots out of his penis.

elective abortion   Termination of a pregnancy by choice, rather than by accident (spontaneous abortion or miscarriage) or in response to an immediate threat to the mother's life (emergency abortion).

embryo   The cells that are produced when the zygote, or fertilized egg, begins to divide; after the seventh week of growth, the embryo becomes a fetus.

Reproductive Rights and Technology

emergency contraception   Also known as the "morning-after pill," though emergency contraception can actually be taken within 72 hours of unprotected intercourse; a series of two hormonal pills that can interrupt the process of fertilization and implantation.

endometrium   Lining of the uterine walls.

enjoin   Legal term meaning "require" or "prohibit"; accomplished through a court order known as an injunction: "The legislature passed a law, but the court enjoined (prohibited) the police from enforcing it."

estrogen   Key female hormone of the menstrual cycle, along with progesterone; synthetic estrogen is used in birth control pills and other treatments of women.

fallopian tube   One of the tubes connecting a woman's ovaries with her uterus; where an egg may be fertilized in unassisted reproduction.

feminist   Believer in the rights of women, particularly someone who believes that women are or have been oppressed and that active resistance to that oppression is needed.

fertility   The ability to create children.

fertility drugs   Medications used to help women become fertile, or able to conceive children. In theory, fertility drugs might be developed for men as well, but so far, none exist. Specifically, fertility drugs are used in controlled ovarian hyperstimulation (COH).

fertilization   Process of a sperm combining with an egg to create potential life; also known as insemination.

fetal anomaly   Something unusual about the fetus, usually a problem that means the fetus cannot survive in utero or will not be able to survive once it is born. A severe fetal anomaly might result in miscarriage (spontaneous abortion); stillbirth (a child being born dead); or the death of the infant soon after birth. Alternately, a child with a severe fetal anomaly might survive but with enormous handicaps.

fetus   Medically speaking, the fertilized egg becomes first an embryo, then, after about seven weeks, when major structures (head, torso, limbs) have been formed, it becomes a fetus. In common speech, *fetus* is often used to refer to the unborn entity from conception through birth.

follicle   Structure within the ovary that contains eggs.

forced sterilization   A procedure that renders a person unable to create children, conducted without that person's consent.

German measles   Rubella, a childhood disease; if a woman is exposed to German measles in her first trimester of pregnancy, the child she is carrying is at grave risk of birth defects.

GIFT (gamete intrafallopian transfer)   A procedure whereby a woman's egg is removed from her body and placed in the fallopian tube of another woman, along with some sperm. Ideally, the sperm will fertilize the egg

142

in the fallopian tube, as happens in unassisted reproduction, and the second woman will become pregnant. The procedure is used to help certain kinds of infertile women.

harvest   To take eggs (or another body part) directly from a person's body. Doctors speak of harvesting the eggs of a woman who is donating eggs or undergoing an in vitro procedure; they also speak of harvesting sperm from men who have died.

higher-order pregnancy   Pregnancy with more than four fetuses; such pregnancies have resulted from the use of ovulation-inducing medication, or fertility drugs, which encourage a woman's body to produce more than one egg. A higher-order pregnancy may also result when several embryos are transferred into a woman's body during an IVF procedure.

Hyde Amendment   The 1977 Congressional bill that banned the use of Medicaid to pay for abortions.

implantation   Process of an embryo attaching itself to uterine walls and then burrowing into the wall, where it grows into a fetus.

impotence   A man's inability to have his penis become erect or stay erect. Impotence and infertility are two different conditions, though an impotent man may have trouble fathering a child. However, a man may be infertile (unable to create children) and still be potent (able to have and sustain an erection).

induced labor   Labor that has been brought on with medication, rather than occurring naturally. Labor may be induced as part of a birthing procedure if the delivery of a woman's child is overdue. It may also be induced as part of a late-term abortion, to help the woman's body expel the fetus. The drug pitocin is most often used to induce labor.

induction   The act of bringing something on. Ovulation induction refers to the process of inducing (bringing on) ovulation, usually with drugs.

infertility   The inability to create children.

informed consent   A legal term referring to a person knowingly giving her or his consent. The term is often used with regard to abortion laws that call for a woman's informed consent to an abortion, in which the law requires a woman to listen to a particular lecture or view certain pictures. Defenders of reproductive rights argue that these kinds of informed consent provisions in abortion laws are really a smokescreen behind which opponents of abortion try to discourage women from having the procedure.

injunction   Legal requirement or prohibition; a doctor might seek an *injunction* against enforcing a law that he or she believes is unconstitutional or medically dangerous.

insemination   Fertilization, whereby sperm enters (inseminates) an egg.

in utero   In the womb.

in vitro   In Latin, literally, "in glass." Used to refer to a procedure that happens in a laboratory (presumably in a glass dish): "The woman's fallopian tube was blocked, so the egg had to be fertilized in vitro," i.e., in a glass dish in a laboratory.

in vitro fertilization (IVF)   A fertility procedure in which a woman's egg is harvested, placed in a glass dish (in vitro), and fertilized with sperm.

judicial bypass or waiver   Legal procedure; with regard to abortion, the term refers to a legal procedure that must be written into any law requiring a minor to inform one or both parents of her intention to have an abortion or to obtain parental consent for an abortion. A judicial bypass or waiver allows the minor to ask a judge to bypass the requirement or have it waived. For example, a judge might rule that it is not in a minor's best interests to tell a particular parent or that the minor cannot locate the parent. The Supreme Court has ruled that any abortion law that involves telling a minor's parents must include a provision for judicial bypass. In fact, several states have passed such laws without provision for judicial bypass, but the Supreme Court has ruled that these laws cannot be enforced.

laparoscopy   Minor surgical procedure performed under general anesthesia in which the doctor inserts instruments through an incision. In fertility medicine, the instruments are inserted into the woman's abdomen in order to view the woman's reproductive organs directly.

majority   More than 50%; when used with regard to Supreme Court decisions, it is contrasted with plurality, which means the largest number but no more than 50%. Since the Supreme Court has nine members, five votes would be a majority but four votes supporting a particular decision might be a plurality—that is, more votes than went to any other single decision.

Medicaid   A government program to fund some kinds of health care for low-income citizens.

menstrual cycle   A nonpregnant woman's sequence of hormonal and chemical events, repeated approximately every month, including menstruation and ovulation. If a woman becomes pregnant, that interrupts her menstrual cycle.

minor   A person under the legal age of adulthood, which is usually 18 but is sometimes 16 or 21.

motile   Able to move; a term used to evaluate sperm (healthy sperm that are capable of fertilization must be motile; sperm that are not motile enough could be a cause of male infertility).

multiple pregnancy   Pregnancy with more than one fetus: twins, triplets, quadruplets, or more.

oocyte   Precursor to eggs; immature egg; also known as germ cell; stored in the follicles.

ovum (singular), **ova** (plural) Egg, eggs.

parental consent A requirement for minors requesting abortions in many states, in which one or both parents or guardians must give written consent before a minor is allowed to have an abortion.

parental notification A requirement for minors requesting abortions in many states, in which one or both parents or guardians must be notified before a minor is allowed to have an abortion.

partial-birth abortion Colloquial term suggesting—inaccurately—that a live child is partially delivered before being terminated. In *Stenberg v. Carhart* (2000), the Supreme Court struck down a Nebraska ban on this type of abortion.

plurality Largest number; when describing Supreme Court decisions, this term is contrasted with majority, which means more than 50%. If four out of nine justices support a particular decision, that may be the largest number of justices to support any one decision—a plurality—while still falling short of a majority (five justices).

potential life Term used in *Roe v. Wade* (1973) to describe the fetus; Supreme Court Justice Harry Blackmun's majority decision referred to "the potential life of the fetus."

preimplantation genetic diagnosis (PGD) Technique used to screen embryos conceived in vitro before the embryos are implanted into a woman's uterus; by removing one of the embryo's eight cells and analyzing it, the doctor has the option of rejecting embryos that carry inherited diseases or have other problems.

pro-choice Term used to indicate people or groups who believe that women should have many reproductive choices, including the right to choose abortion.

progestin Any synthetic compound that mimics progesterone (a female hormone) by maintaining the thickness of the endometrium. Progestin is used in oral contraceptives, emergency contraception, and other hormonal treatments of women.

progesterone Key female hormone in the menstrual cycle, along with estrogen; used in oral contraception, emergency contraception, and other hormonal treatments of women.

pro-life Term used to indicate people or groups who believe that abortion is murder and should not be allowed or should be allowed only under extreme circumstances. Some (though not all) pro-life advocates would permit abortion to save the life of the woman, or in cases of rape or incest.

pronucleus Zygote; an egg that has been fertilized but has not yet undergone cell division.

quickening Old-fashioned term for the fetus's beginning to move, as experienced by the pregnant woman. Quickening usually takes place in the fourth or fifth month. In English common law (the basis for much U.S. law) and in early U.S. law and custom, abortions performed before quickening were not generally considered either illegal or immoral.

rhythm method   Periodic abstinence or FAMs (Fertility Awareness Methods); a method of birth control that consists of only having intercourse on the days when a woman is not ovulating, on the theory that only on those days can she become pregnant. However, studies have shown that ovulation can be induced unexpectedly by a number of factors, including sexual intercourse.

right to life   Term used to indicate a central idea of the anti-abortion movement: that the fetus has a right to life. Pro-life organizations or politicians may also be referred to as being "right-to-life."

Roe v. Wade   Landmark 1973 Supreme Court decision holding that a woman's right to choose abortion was protected under the Fourteenth Amendment without reservations in the first trimester. Starting in the second trimester, the State may regulate abortion with the goal of protecting women's health; starting in the third trimester, the State may regulate abortion with the goal of protecting "the potential life of the fetus."

RU-486   Mifepristone, a pill that, taken with misoprostol, can induce an abortion in a woman up to seven weeks pregnant. Long available in Europe, this medication was only recently approved for U.S. use by the FDA.

semen   Fluid containing sperm, ejaculated by men during orgasm.

singleton   Single fetus; as opposed to multiple fetuses: twins, triplets, quadruplets, or more.

speculum   Instrument that holds open a woman's vagina, used during gynecological exams and procedures, when the doctor or staff person needs to either examine the woman's vagina and/or cervix; take a sample from either body part; or insert something into the woman's vagina, cervix, or uterus. Women have also used speculums and mirrors to examine themselves.

sperm   Men's contribution to the genetic process; male sex cells, produced in the testes.

sperm bank   Facility where men can sell or donate sperm and women can purchase sperm. Women whose husbands are infertile or who do not have male partners may wish to become pregnant with sperm from a sperm bank. Many sperm banks have policies limiting access to their services to married women.

sperm washing   A treatment that removes all the components from the semen except the sperm, to make the sperm more highly concentrated and thus more likely to fertilize an egg.

spermicide   Chemical compound that immobilizes sperm.

Glossary

State   Legal term referring both to the government of an individual state and to government in general.

sterility   Infertility, being unable to create children.

sterilization   Surgical or other procedure that results in the person being unable to create children.

surrogate mother   Literally, "substitute mother"; used to refer to a woman pregnant with a baby that she intends to give to another woman who will be the child's legal mother. A surrogate may be carrying a child created with one of her own eggs, or with an egg implanted from another woman.

trimester   Period representing one-third; the 39–40 weeks of pregnancy are divided into three periods known as trimesters. The first trimester lasts for 13 weeks; the second runs from week 14 to week 24; the third trimester begins in week 25 and continues until birth.

tubal pregnancy   See *ectopic pregnancy*.

ultrasound   Sonogram, a procedure by which sonar is used to view the fetus within the woman's womb.

unassisted reproduction   "Natural" reproduction; the creation of a child without the assistance of drugs, surgery, IVF, ART, or any other medical technology.

unemancipated minor   Someone too young to be considered a legal adult, for whom a parent, guardian, or state institution is responsible. In contrast, an emancipated minor is a young person legally allowed adult responsibilities, for whom no one is responsible. Even in states where minors are required to obtain parental consent or to notify their parents of their intention to have an abortion, an emancipated minor can have an abortion without parental notification or consent.

uterus   Womb; the female organ in which an embryo is implanted and where a fetus grows.

viable   Feasible, possible; the word used to describe fetuses that are able to survive outside the womb, which usually occurs around week 25 of the pregnancy.

zona pellucida   Clear covering surrounding the egg, which must be penetrated by a sperm for fertilization to occur.

zygote   Fertilized egg, pronucleus.

PART II

GUIDE TO FURTHER RESEARCH

CHAPTER 6

HOW TO RESEARCH REPRODUCTIVE RIGHTS AND TECHNOLOGY

One of the biggest challenges faced by the researcher of reproductive rights and technology is the rapidly changing nature of both topics. Reproductive technology is a field in which new medical research and innovative fertility treatments are continually being announced. The political landscape of reproductive rights is constantly shifting (although certain trends can be identified). A book on either topic with a copyright date of more than two years ago must be viewed with caution if not suspicion, for it is likely that much of the material is not only out of date but misleadingly so. Even newspaper or magazine articles are less useful than they might be for another topic; a popular article on cloning, for example, will be out of date almost before it is published, while a newspaper story on reproductive rights may focus on an issue—such as RU-486 or stem-cell research—whose outcome remains uncertain for months at a time.

A second problem is the widely divergent views that characterize both fields. In the area of reproductive technology, there are those who greet the new scientific developments with excitement, those who see them as doomsday warnings, and those who express every possible response in between. Even religious leaders, legal experts, and political analysts confess themselves baffled by the ethical, legal, and social issues raised by new fertility treatments and the latest scientific capabilities. In reproductive rights, there are an enormous number of ethical and political positions that cannot adequately be summed up by the terms *pro-life* and *pro-choice*. Moreover, both the pro-life and the pro-choice movements are part of larger movements with complicated political agendas—agendas that may or may not be shared by the rank-and-file activists in each movement. Thus researchers in both fields must be careful not to rely upon a single article or book without having at least some idea of how its author might join in the various debates raging about these topics.

Reproductive Rights and Technology

A third problem concerns the technical nature of both fields—and the way that people's politics shapes their discussion of apparently objective fact. For example, most fertility treatments focus on procedures that affect women far more than men. The man may masturbate to contribute sperm, while the woman undergoes a complicated hormonal regime followed by the process of egg retrieval and/or implantation with a fertilized egg or embryo. It would not necessarily be clear, from a treatment's description, that the procedure might have been developed to cope with male infertility, as a way of insuring that poor quality sperm was given every possible aid in fertilizing an egg. The beginning researcher, reading the scientific information, might easily assume that infertility was a primarily female problem, given that the most advanced science focuses on female bodies. The researcher must be continually ready to ask the big questions: "How often is this treatment successful? How painful is it? How does it affect the feelings of the woman and the man involved? What are the possible side effects for the woman? For the child? Who can afford it? Is it worth it? Why or why not?" These questions are rarely asked when fertility treatments are being described, yet they are fundamental to our understanding of reproductive technology and its effects on our society.

Likewise, when reading about reproductive rights, the researcher might easily be misled or confused by the highly divergent language used by each side. Pro-choice activists talk about "procedures"; pro-life activists refer to "murders." Pro-choice activists talk about "the fetus"; pro-life activists talk about "the unborn child." The term "partial-birth abortion," coined by pro-life activists, is considered misleading and inflammatory by those who support abortion rights; the pro-life movement, for its part, considers the language of abortion rights to be misleadingly clinical and impersonal. The researcher who comes across articles, editorials, and opinion pieces by or about people on either side of the issue might easily assume that there was, indeed, only one accepted way of talking about abortion or might mistake a politically biased description for objective scientific fact. Researchers looking at reproductive rights must be familiar with the language and approaches of both sides, so that they can evaluate everything they read, even material that would seem to be straightforward and factual.

Finally, researchers into reproductive rights and/or technology must be aware of their own biases, their own assumptions about women, men, families, science, and society. Is there a "natural" way of birth that science ought not to interfere with, or should our society welcome scientific advances in fertility the way most people have welcomed vaccinations and antibiotics? How important is biology to being a parent? Does it really matter whose eggs and sperm created a particular child? Does it matter in whose womb the child develops? Is a legal contract more important than a physical relationship? Is donating egg and sperm more important than the nine-month experience of carrying a child? Are children meant to be taken as they come, or is it our responsibility to shape them as far as we can? Do men and women have "natural" relationships to sexuality and parenting, or are these relationships socially constructed, or both? And, are we happy with the ways that women and men have traditionally related to their sexuality and their bodies, or are we interested in opening up new arenas that might support new kinds of behavior and relationships? What is the relationship between the nuclear family and our society? What should that relationship be?

Clearly, there are no easy answers to these questions. It may even be difficult to identify that each of us holds some opinion on all of them, whether we have thought about it consciously or not. Yet without becoming aware of these underlying questions and choosing a conscious response to them, we cannot hope to make the political decisions called for by the challenging fields of reproductive rights and reproductive technology. Moreover, for research to be effective, researchers must be aware of their own feelings and thoughts about these issues. Otherwise, certain responses will seem "obvious" or "natural" to the researcher—while not being shared by his or her audience. Certain facts, opinions, and political developments will seem to need no explanation or to "go without saying"—an attitude that is hardly conducive to good research.

How, then, can researchers proceed? Here are some general suggestions, followed by more specific advice about where to find material.

TIPS FOR RESEARCHING REPRODUCTIVE RIGHTS

- **Define the topic as specifically as possible.** Whether surfing the Net, looking through a bookstore, exploring a library, or doing a database search, one is likely to run into an overwhelming amount of material, even on an apparently narrowly defined topic. It is helpful for researchers to know exactly what questions they are asking and to have some idea of what would count as a complete answer. Even as narrowly defined a topic as the RU-486 controversy has many facets: several years of history as pro-choice and pro-life groups battle over the pill; contrasting responses from different presidential administrations; the biology of how the pill works; the European experience; the pro-choice argument that the pill will make abortion a more private matter and less accessible to the clinic protests and legal restrictions that the right-to-life movement has employed; the pro-life argument that women using the "abortion pill" experience devastating psychological consequences for which they are not prepared; the argument over how much specialized knowledge a doctor ought to have to prescribe the pill; and many other issues. The researcher who wants to find out about RU-486 and is not prepared to decide—either ahead of time or during the search—just which aspect of the topic is most important, is likely to be buried under a mound of contradictory facts and conflicting opinions.

- **Do not settle for easy answers.** On the other hand, it is all too easy to see reproductive rights topics as far simpler than they really are. A researcher into the RU-486 controversy who focused only on the science would miss the political dimensions of this debate. Why are pro-life groups so adamantly opposed to the pill, and why do pro-choice groups see it as so important? How has RU-486 been treated differently than Viagra? Exactly how does the pill work? (In fact, it is actually two pills.) It can be hard to strike a balance between making a topic overly narrow and allowing it to become overly broad—but this balancing act is exactly what is needed when exploring reproductive rights.

- **Be aware of the historical landmarks.** Of course, the story of reproductive rights is contradictory and complicated and cannot simply be summed up with a few dates. But having a few dates in mind can help clarify the issues, enabling the researcher to identify the context in which a particular event takes place. Among the most important landmarks in the modern reproductive rights movements are the FDA approval of oral contraception in 1960; the *Roe v. Wade* decision of 1973; the passage of the Hyde Amendment in 1977; the election of Ronald Reagan in 1980; the beginning of the rescue movement in the late 1980s; the Supreme Court's *Webster* decision in 1989; the Supreme Court's *Planned Parenthood v. Casey* decision in 1992; the clinic violence of the mid-1990s; the Supreme Court decision *Stenberg v. Carhart* in 2000; the FDA approval of mifepristone (RU-486) in 2000; and the pro-life appointments of George W. Bush in early 2001.

- **Know the source.** Widely divergent opinions exist on virtually every aspect of reproductive rights. Some people support making contraception widely available but oppose abortion. Some people see providing condoms to teenagers as anathema but willingly support public funding for sterilization of women on welfare. Some people see abortion rights issues as primarily about the family, or society, or women's sexuality; other people see the decision to have an abortion as intensely private and object to any political group putting the issue into a larger context. It would be possible to continue listing diverse opinions on reproductive rights, which is far too complicated to be summed up as merely "pro-choice" vs. "pro-life." On the other hand, sometimes that simple, two-part distinction is all that matters, as people rush to line up on one side or the other. Knowing who is writing (or being interviewed or quoted), what the context is, and why a person might focus on a particular point is extremely important for the researcher.

TIPS FOR RESEARCHING
REPRODUCTIVE TECHNOLOGY

- **Know the science.** Certainly, it is possible to research this topic without having an advanced degree in science; most reporters covering the issue probably have no more than a B.A. in the liberal arts. But without a basic sense of how reproduction works and of how women's reproductive systems operate, it is virtually impossible to follow the medical descriptions of new treatments and research. Most newspapers and general-interest magazines will explain the new treatments in fairly simple terms, but they assume a basic knowledge of anatomy and biology.

- **Keep a sense of perspective.** Often, a fertility treatment will be heralded by a news story whose headline suggests that every doctor in the country will be offering the procedure tomorrow, with a 100% success rate. Yet many of the innovations reported in both the general and the scientific press are highly experimental. They may be simply ideas that a scientist is exploring, the one-time results of an experiment that worked, or a procedure that has been successful with only a small, select handful of women. Moreover, news reports of scientific developments tend to downplay the downside: the side effects, the failure rates, the costs, the psychological toll that a test might take on a woman, a man, or a relationship. On the other hand, scientific developments are sometimes treated as doomsday scenarios by reporters or columnists who see a brave new world filled with cloned slaves and genetic overlords behind every report of a scientific advance. Researchers who keep their own sense of perspective will do a better job of evaluating just how significant a new development might be.

- **Know the debates.** Developments in reproductive technology have inspired a range of debates about legal, ethical, and social issues. Being familiar with these debates, and asking how people on various sides might view a particular scientific achievement, can help a researcher put information into perspective.

GETTING STARTED:
HOW TO FIND HELPFUL SOURCES

BOOKS

Reproductive Rights

Researchers must of course consult libraries and bookstores for the latest publications on this topic, since the field is changing so constantly. A few basic history books, however, are still considered the best in the field. The "grandmother" of reproductive rights books is Linda Gordon's *Woman's Body. Woman's Right: A Social History of Birth Control in America* (New York: Penguin, 1977). This classic feminist history of the fight for contraceptive rights in pre-1975 America argues that women's ability to control their own reproduction was a central part of the fight for women's liberation. Gordon also explores the ways in which nineteenth-century feminists saw birth control as threatening, because it seemed to them that if women could control their own reproduction, men would be given carte blanche to sexually exploit women. Readers looking for an overview of how birth control and abortion were viewed in the days before *Roe v. Wade* would do well to start with Gordon's classic work.

A useful supplement to Gordon's account is Ellen Chesler's *Woman of Valor: Margaret Sanger and the Birth Control Movement in America* (New York: Simon & Schuster, 1992). This admiring but critical biography of Margaret Sanger conveys an excellent sense of the various social opinions that came into play as Sanger tried different strategies to win acceptance for contraception.

Readers looking for insight into the worldviews and motivations of both pro-choice and pro-life women can find an excellent source in Faye D. Ginsburg's *Contested Lives: The Abortion Debate in an American Community* (updated edition with a new introduction; Berkeley and Los Angeles: Berkeley: University of California Press, 1998). Ginsburg, a New York anthropologist, went to Fargo, North Dakota, in the mid-1980s to conduct this groundbreaking study of the battle over a local women's health clinic. Ginsburg takes the Fargo experience as emblematic of conflicts throughout the nation. She does an effective job in portraying what each political position feels like "from the inside" and then steps back and places both sides in a larger context.

The volumes just discussed have all been primarily pro-choice. There are far fewer academic overviews of the topic from the pro-life perspective; the classic texts in that field have tended to be written for a broader audience, published by religious rather than academic or mainstream presses. A major exception is John Noonan's *A Private Choice: Abortion in America in the Seventies* (New York: Free Press, 1979), in which the distinguished Catholic jurist analyzes the issue of abortion after *Roe v. Wade* and offers a philosophical and legal basis for opposing abortion. Noonan's book is more than 20 years old, but the arguments he advances still hold power for the pro-life movement.

Another way of gaining access to the pro-life perspective is through the autobiographical accounts of Norma McCorvey and Bernard Nathanson. McCorvey's book tells of her own experience as the pseudonymous "Roe" in *Roe v. Wade* and chronicles her journey from abortion rights activist to pro-life born-again Christian (with Gary Thomas, *Won by Love: Norma McCorvey, Jane Roe of Roe v. Wade, Speaks Out for the Unborn as She Shares her New Conviction for Life*, Nashville, Tenn.: Thomas Nelson, 1998). Bernard Nathanson helped found the National Association for the Repeal of Abortion Laws (NARAL); he was also the director of the then-largest abortion facility in the world. He then became certain that life begins at conception, joined the pro-life movement, and eventually converted to Catholicism, a series of experiences that he describes in *The Hand of God: A Journey from Death to Life by the Abortion Doctor Who Changed His Mind* (Washington, D.C.: Regnery Publishing, 1996). Both McCorvey's and Nathanson's accounts have been criticized as inaccurate by people who participated with them in pro-choice movements, but McCorvey's story, in particular, provides an inside view of the pro-choice and feminist movements, as McCorvey accuses both movements of being dominated by upper-middle-class women who ignored and marginalized her.

Researchers looking for basic factual information on reproductive rights might begin with NARAL's yearly volume *Who Decides? A State-by-State Review of Abortion and Reproductive Rights*. This detailed overview contains information on each state's reproductive rights law; the positions of governors, state legislatures, and the major political parties; and a list of pro-life and pro-choice legislative measures enacted in the past year. Although NARAL is of course strongly pro-choice, the basic legal information will be of use to people on all sides of the issue.

Basic legal information is also available in Maureen Harrison and Steve Gilbert's three-volume work, *Abortion Decisions of the United States Supreme Court, Vol. 1, the 1970s; Vol. II, the 1980s; Vol. III, the 1990s* (Beverly Hills, Calif.: Excellent Books, 1993). Each volume includes copies of a decade's worth of U.S. Supreme Court decisions on abortion, from *Roe v. Wade* (1973) through *Bray v. Alexandria Women's Health Clinic* (1993), edited for the lay reader: Legal terminology has been explained in brackets, extensive citations have been removed, and each decision is introduced with a one-page summary and a list of the justices then on the Court. The first two volumes also have statistics on the number of abortions performed each year of the decade; each volume has a copy of the U.S. Constitution for easy reference in the back.

Reproductive Technology

Because this field is constantly changing, researchers run the constant risk that anything they read will be out of date before they have finished. Authors, rather than titles, are probably of use here. Researchers might begin by finding the latest volumes by the following writers, while examining earlier works to see if they are still relevant:

- Lori Andrews is a legal expert on reproductive technology who has been personally involved as an advisor or attorney on many key cases in the field over the last two decades. She has become extremely critical of the field she helped to develop, and her works combine her vast personal experience with her legal knowledge and ethical responses.
- Roger Gosden is a pioneering embryologist who writes enthusiastically about the latest developments in reproductive technology. He, too, has inside experience as a scientist who continues to work in the field.
- Gina Kolata has been the science reporter for the *New York Times* for several years. She covered the story of Dolly, the first large mammal ever cloned, and wrote a book-length account of Dolly's story. She continues to write on science issues.
- Gregory Pence is a medical ethicist and philosopher who writes sympathetically and calmly about cloning, raising questions about the doomsday scenarios that the topic seems to inspire, and calling for a more balanced view of what he sees as exciting scientific developments. His focus is on the human implications of the scientific advances.

For researchers who are seeking the latest basic information on fertility treatments, two major organizations—RESOLVE and the American Society of Reproductive Medicine (ASRM)—have recently published books. However, by the time this volume goes to press, new and more up-to-date works will probably be on the market. Researchers are encouraged to search for the most recently published books on fertility aids, looking carefully at the authors' credentials. (Sandra Ann Carson, M.D., Peter R. Casson, M.D., and Deborah J. Shuman's *The American Society for Reproductive Medicine: Complete Guide to Fertility* [Lincolnwood, IL: Contemporary Books, 1999] was used to help prepare this book.)

NEWSPAPERS AND MAGAZINES

One excellent way to research reproductive rights and technology is to pick a topic—either broad or narrow—and do a database search, deciding in advance how far back in time the search will go. In preparing this book, ProQuest, the database used by the New York Public Library, was very helpful, but many others are available. Most databases will provide both an abstract and the full article; however, because of a recently settled lawsuit, the *New York Times* provides only abstracts free of charge for anything published before December 1999. Other periodicals have followed the *Times*'s example and have begun instituting a fee for examining or printing a full article.

Some useful key words for searches are *reproductive rights, abortion, pro-life, pro-choice, right-to-life; reproductive technology, fertility,* and *infertility.* Because each of these topics will turn up a huge number of articles, narrower topics may be more useful, but certainly any one of these key terms will help researchers gain an overview of activity in the past year.

A useful approach to researching reproductive rights is to choose a periodical or an author that expresses a particular point of view, so as to find out how the pro-choice or pro-life movements are analyzing a particular event. It may also be useful to read particular writers as a way of tracking the general political climate. Here are some suggestions:

- **Useful pro-choice periodicals:** *The Humanist, Ms., The Nation, National NOW Times, The Village Voice*

- **Useful pro-life periodicals:** *America, Christianity Today, Human Life Review, National Catholic Reporter, National Review*

- **Useful pro-choice commentators:** Ellen Goodman, Katha Pollitt, Ellen Willis

- **Useful pro-life commentators:** Harry J. Byrne, Richard J. Goldkamp, George F. Will

RESEARCH AND THE INTERNET

The Internet can be an invaluable resource for the researcher on reproductive rights and technology: to locate a court case, get background on a key figure, find out the latest news on a particular topic, or access a scientific explanation.

The search engine Google (http://www.google.com) is a particularly effective way of answering specific questions or locating specific information on reproductive rights and technology. Searches conducted in the course of writing this book turned up information as diverse as a law review article on forced sterilization, a brief history of birth control, several contemporary articles on clinic violence, a listing of all Supreme Court cases involving abortion or contraception, and profiles of pro-life leaders Joseph Scheidler, Randall Terry, and Antonin Scalia. Researchers looking to read a wide range of opinions on a topic or to quickly find the "pro-life" or "pro-choice" position on a particular issue can easily meet their needs on the Net. Indeed, because of the fast-changing nature of the topics, the Internet is a useful place to find the information that can not yet have been published in book form. Be careful: Often, information on the Net is not marked with a date, and a researcher can easily find out-of-date information without realizing it.

The Planned Parenthood web site (http://www.plannedparenthood.org) is probably the single most useful source of information for those interested in reproductive rights and technology, with legal information about court decisions, scientific explanations of contraception, and many links to other sites. Although Planned Parenthood is a pro-choice organization, much of the information on this site will be useful even to those who do not share the group's perspective. The site includes abortion information, a listing and analysis of Supreme Court decisons, and information about teen pregnancy.

The Ultimate Pro-Life Resource List (http://www.prolifeinfo.org) bills itself as "the most comprehensive listing of right-to-life resources on the Internet" and it seems to live up to its billing; however, since the site strongly opposes abortion-related violence, it does not include such groups in its listing. With that exception, the site has links to a huge range of pro-life groups, including national organizations, state groups, local organizations, college groups, Canadian organizations, international organizations, groups related to political parties, organizations that oppose euthanasia, health-related groups, abortion alternatives, post-abortion counseling and information, and religious groups.

Researchers looking for specific court cases and legislation can turn to one of the many free sources for legal information on the web. Unfortunately, electronic law libraries—including Westlaw and Lexis-Nexis—all charge fees for use, either via subscription or on a per-use basis, and they are the only really reliable way to get comprehensive online access to court cases before 1990, other than Supreme Court cases, which are readily available through Findlaw (http://findlaw.com) and the Legal Information Institute (http://lii.cornell.edu). Findlaw also offers a comprehensive directory of various Internet legal resources, including a state-by-state guide, while the Legal Information Insititute offers pages that focus on "educational policy," "employment policy," and "discrimination law." Be aware that many states do not offer online texts of court cases; many others go back only a few years or, at most, to 1990.

Another useful Internet resource is the Meta-Index for U.S. Legal Research, a service of Georgia State University's College of Law: http://gsu-law.gsu.edu.metaindex. You can access Supreme Court cases, circuit court cases, federal legislation, and federal regulations, as well as find links to other online law resources. Cornell Law School's Legal Information Institute (http://law.cornell.edu) also offers a variety of legal resources. This site is extremely useful for obtaining Supreme Court information.

CHAPTER 7

ANNOTATED BIBLIOGRAPHY

The following bibliography contains three major sections: books, articles, and web sites. The books and articles sections are divided into two parts: reproductive rights and reproductive technology. Because many web sites contain information on both topics, they are simply presented alphabetically.

The books section is by no means a comprehensive listing of all of the books on this wide-ranging topic. Rather, it is an effort to give an overview of the topics of reproductive rights and reproductive technology, offering some important, representative volumes that a beginning researcher might find useful. Researchers should be aware of how quickly books in this field go out of date. In reproductive technology, new scientific developments are taking place daily, while in reproductive rights, the nation's political climate changes almost as fast. This listing is therefore designed to help the beginning researcher grasp the kinds of books that ought to be consulted. Included are some historical works; major writings by key figures on all sides of the debates; and books describing the latest political and scientific debates.

The articles were drawn primarily from newspapers and general-interest magazines, with some articles from political and opinion journals on all sides of the issues, and some specialized journals in law, ethics, science, and the social sciences. Most of the articles listed here are accessible to the general reader with no specialized knowledge; some of the "specialized journal" listings require more background.

The web sites here likewise do not represent the virtual universe of available Internet resources. They do, however, constitute a good starting place for the beginning researcher, along with an assurance that with these listings, the researcher can begin to keep up with major political, legal, and scientific events in the ever-changing field of reproductive rights and technology.

Annotated Bibliography

Annotated Bibliography

BOOKS

REPRODUCTIVE RIGHTS

Andrusko, Dave, ed. *To Rescue the Future: The Pro-Life Movement in the 1980's.* Harrison, N.Y.: Life Cycle Press, 1983. An anthology of articles representing the concerns of the pro-life movement. Useful for providing opinions on a wide range of concerns, including such issues as how the press presents pro-life activists, as well as more personal responses to abortion.

Baehr, Ninia. *Abortion Without Apology: A Radical History for the 1990s.* Boston: South End Press, 1990. A strong defense of abortion and reproductive choice, offering an historical perspective as well as a political argument.

Chen, Constance M. *"The Sex Side of Life": Mary Ware Dennett's Pioneering Battle for Birth Control and Sex Education.* New York: New Press, 1996. A biography of Mary Ware Dennett, a pioneering birth-control crusader who was first a colleague, then a rival, of Margaret Sanger. This book offers a critical view of Sanger as dictatorial and overly conciliatory to the medical establishment, while portraying in a more positive light Dennett's view that women, not doctors, should control their own contraceptive decisions.

Chesler, Ellen. *Woman of Valor: Margaret Sanger and the Birth Control Movement in America.* New York: Simon & Schuster, 1992. An admiring but critical biography of Margaret Sanger, the pioneering leader of the early U.S. movement for birth control.

Chesler, Phyllis. *Sacred Bond: The Legacy of Baby M.* New York: First Vintage Books, 1988. A feminist looks at the Baby M case, in which a long legal battle resulted in a judge finally awarding custody of a child to the child's father, rather than to her biological mother. Chesler argues that only in a patriarchal society could a woman's experience of pregnancy and attachment to the child she had carried be viewed as less valuable than a father's sperm donation and a legal contract.

Faludi, Susan. *Backlash: The Undeclared War Against American Women.* New York: Crown, 1991. Faludi argues that the media's misreporting of major stories contributed to the pressures on women to conform to traditional roles during the 1980s. She focuses particularly on the fertility scare and one news story that she claims was used in a particularly inaccurate way.

Garton, Jean Staker. *Who Broke the Baby?* Minneapolis, Minn.: Bethany House, 1998. A classic pro-life text in a new edition. Garton uses a Christian perspective to examine pro-choice slogans, arguing that such phrases

163

as "A woman has a right to control her own body," "Every child a wanted child," and "A fetus is not a person," are euphemistic and untrue.

Ginsburg, Faye D. *Contested Lives: The Abortion Debate in an American Community*. Updated edition with a new introduction. Berkeley and Los Angeles: University of California Press, 1998. A groundbreaking portrait of the battle over a women's health clinic in Fargo, North Dakota, taking the Fargo experience as emblematic of conflicts between pro-choice and pro-life women in the 1980s.

Gordon, Linda. *Woman's Body, Woman's Right: A Social History of Birth Control in America*. New York: Penguin, 1977. The classic feminist history of the fight for contraceptive rights in pre-1975 America. Gordon argues that women's ability to control their own reproduction was a central part of the fight for women's liberation but also points out that women, too, fought to suppress birth control as one way of protecting themselves from men's sexual advances and to hold men responsible for their own sexual behavior.

Hardon, Anita, and Elizabeth Hayes, eds. *Reproductive Rights in Practice: A Feminist Report on the Quality of Care*. New York: Zed Books, 1997. A volume compiled by the Women's Health Action Foundation, a group dedicated to improving women's health worldwide "by encouraging the rational use of drugs and promoting the improvement of health services available to women"; the study contains an overview of family planning programs in eight countries: Nigeria, Kenya, Bolivia, Mexico, Bangladesh, Thailand, Finland, and the Netherlands.

Harrison, Maureen, and Steve Gilbert, eds. *Abortion Decisions of the United States Supreme Court, Vol. I, the 1970s; Vol. II, the 1980s; Vol. III, the 1990s*. Beverly Hills, Calif.: Excellent Books, 1993. Copies of each U.S. Supreme Court decisions on abortion, from *Roe v. Wade* (1973) through *Bray v. Alexandria Women's Health Clinic* (1993), edited for the lay reader: Legal terminology has been explained in brackets, extensive citations have been removed, and each decision is introduced with a one-page summary and a list of the justices then on the Court. The first two volumes also have statistics on the number of abortions performed each year of the decade; each volume has a copy of the U.S. Constitution for easy reference in the back.

McCorvey, Norma, and Gary Thomas. *Won by Love: Norma McCorvey, Jane Roe of Roe v. Wade, Speaks Out for the Unborn as She Shares her New Conviction for Life*. Nashville, Tenn.: Thomas Nelson, 1998. An account of the experiences of Norma McCorvey, the anonymous "Roe" of *Roe v. Wade*. McCorvey spent years working for abortion rights, but she felt disrespected by her feminist colleagues and loved by the Operation Rescue pro-life protestors at the clinic where she worked. Eventually, she became a pro-life activist and a religious Christian, a journey chronicled in this book.

NARAL (National Abortion and Reproductive Rights Action League) and NARAL Foundation. *Who Decides? A State-by-State Review of Abortion and Reproductive Rights.* Tenth edition, NARAL, 2001. A single volume, updated yearly, that contains detailed information on each state's reproductive rights law regarding abortion, contraception, and other reproductive rights issues. In addition to describing the legal situation in each state, the volume includes the positions of governors and state legislatures on choice, positions of major political parties on a woman's right to choose abortion, and a list of anti- and pro-choice legislative measures enacted in the past year. Although NARAL is of course strongly pro-choice, the basic legal information will be of use to people on all sides of the issue.

Nathanson, Bernard. *The Hand of God: A Journey from Death to Life by the Abortion Doctor Who Changed His Mind.* Washington, D.C.; Regnery Publishing, 1996. A story of the life and work of Bernard Nathanson, one of the major leaders of the pro-life movement and the producer/narrator of *The Silent Scream*, a video that purports to show an abortion through the use of ultrasound. In 1968, Nathanson was a co-founder of the National Association for the Repeal of Abortion Laws (NARAL); he was also the director of the then-largest abortion facility in the world. He then became certain that life begins at conception, joined the pro-life movement, and eventually converted to Catholicism. He describes these experiences in this book.

Noonan, John. *A Private Choice: Abortion in America in the Seventies.* New York: Free Press, 1979. The distinguished Catholic jurist analyzes the issue of abortion after *Roe v. Wade*, offering a philosophical and legal basis for opposing abortion.

Petchesky, Rosalind P., and Karen Judd, eds. *Negotiating Reproductive Rights: Women's Perspectives Across Countries and Cultures.* New York: Zed Books, 1998. This book features studies of reproductive rights in seven countries: Brazil, Egypt, Malaysia, Mexico, Nigeria, the Philippines, and the United States (U.S. information focuses on the experiences of women of color).

Pollitt, Katha. *Reasonable Creatures: Essays on Women and Feminism.* New York: Vintage Books, 1995. This collection of feminist essays by a *Nation* columnist takes on a wide range of issues, including the battle over Baby M, the notion of fetal rights, and abortion rights. A strong pro-choice advocate, Pollitt's essays offer a topical perspective on those issues as seen in the mid-1990s.

———. *Subject to Debate: Sense and Dissents on Women, Politics, and Culture.* New York: Modern Library, 2001. A collection of columns that Pollitt

165

wrote for *The Nation* on contemporary politics, with a strong focus on reproductive rights issues, including abortion and RU-486.

Reagan, Leslie J. *When Abortion Was a Crime: Women, Medicine, and Law in the United States, 1867–1973.* Berkeley: University of California Press, 1977. A look at the history of abortion and the ways that it affected U.S. women.

Scheidler, Joseph. *Closed: 99 Ways to Stop Abortion.* Tan Books & Publishers, Inc., 1994. A pro-life movement classic that first appeared in 1985 as part of the "rescue" movement's efforts to shut down abortion clinics and use civil disobedience tactics to prevent women from having abortions. Although not as popular as in the mid-1980s, the book is still being used today.

Williams, Joan. *Gender Wars: Selfless Women in the Republic of Choice.* New York: NYU Press, 1991. Williams argues that women who choose abortion are actually making a loving and responsible—even a maternal—choice, which is not captured by current pro-choice rhetoric. She advises feminists to communicate stories of "good mothers" who choose to have an abortion, perhaps to meet the needs of a handicapped child or to better care for the children they already have.

Willis, Ellen. *No More Nice Girls: Countercultural Essays.* Middletown, Conn.: Wesleyan University Press, 1994. A feminist analysis of a variety of issues, including abortion and reproductive rights. Willis is known for her commitment to women's pleasure and for the argument that women's sexual pleasure and sexual freedom must be a central part of any kind of women's liberation.

REPRODUCTIVE TECHNOLOGY

Aaronson, Diane, and RESOLVE. *Resolving Infertility: Understanding the Options and Choosing Solutions When You Want to Have a Baby.* New York: Harper Resource, 1999. A resource put together by RESOLVE, an organization founded in 1974 to provide information and emotional and legislative support for people who cannot have children; a thorough guide to medical treatments and other options for responding to infertility.

Andrews, Lori B. *The Clone Age: Adventures in the New World of Reproductive Technology.* With a new afterword. New York: Henry Holt, 2000. An extremely readable, personal, and fact-filled account of the last two decades of developments in reproductive technology, written by a legal expert who was herself involved in many of the decisions and developments as they emerged.

———. *Future Perfect.* New York: Columbia University Press, 2001. Andrews continues her research from *The Clone Age* in this incisive look at

166

the ethical and legal problems raised by the new reproductive technologies, offering suggestions for how regulations and other protections might be put in place.

Annas, George J. *Some Choice: Law, Medicine, and the Market.* New York: Oxford University Press, 1998. A major legal expert on reproductive technology offers his critique of the commercialization of U.S. medicine and the moral dilemmas that this market orientation raises for doctors, patients, and society at large; much of the book has appeared as "Legal Issues in Medicine" articles in the prestigious *New England Journal of Medicine.*

Baker, Robin. *Sex in the Future: The Reproductive Revolution and How It Will Change Us.* New York: Arcade, 2000. The author argues that "The demise of the nuclear familiy is an inevitable step in social evolution," as IVF, surrogate motherhood, cloning, and other technological advances make traditional families obsolete. A strikingly positive view of the potential of reproductive technology.

Barbiere, Robert L., M.D., et al. *Six Steps to Increased Fertility: An Integrated Mind/Body and Medical Program to Promote Conception.* New York: Simon & Schuster, 2000. A guide to fertility that integrates both natural and medical approaches.

Becker, Gay. *The Elusive Embryo: How Men and Women Approach New Reproductive Technologies.* Berkeley: University of California, 2000. Becker argues that infertility is no longer a neutral term but is now perceived as a disease that needs to be cured. Her study of more than 300 women and men has led her to conclude that infertility treatments are being made to look deceptively safe and successful, as well as morally necessary, although in fact, she argues, women undergoing the techniques feel dehumanized while men tend to feel left out.

Buchanan, Allen, Dan W. Brock, Norman Daniels, and Daniel Wikler. *From Chance to Choice: Genetics and Justice.* Cambridge, U.K.: Cambridge University Press, 2000. An exploration of some of the ethical and legal dilemmas that may arise from the new reproductive technologies.

Carson, Sandra Ann, M.D., and Peter R. Casson, M.D., with Deborah J. Shuman. *The American Society for Reproductive Medicine: Complete Guide to Fertility.* Lincolnwood, Ill.: Contemporary Books, 1999. The official guide to the latest information on fertility treatments (as of 1999) by the major U.S. organization of doctors specializing in such treatments.

Clarke, Adele E. *Disciplining Reproduction: Modernity, American Life Sciences and the Problems of Sex.* Berkeley: University of California Press, 1998. A study of how reproductive science developed from 1910 to 1963, analyzing the field as part of the modern drive for control over nature and the search for universal laws.

Cole-Turner, Ronald, ed. *Human Cloning: Religious Responses*. Louisville, Ky.: Westminster John Knox Press, 1997. A collection of essays responding to cloning and reproductive technologies from a religious perspective.

Colker, Ruth. *Pregnant Men: Practice, Theory, and the Law*. Bloomington, Ind.: Indiana University Press, 1994. If men could get pregnant, too, Colker argues, we could formulate a theory of equality that applied equally well to both men and women. As there are no pregnant men, Colker examines instead men who are in similar situations to pregnant women—and shows that they are systematically treated better than women.

Daniels, K., and E. Haimes, eds. *Donor Insemination: International Perspectives*, Cambridge, England: Cambridge University Press, 1998. The first collection of essays viewing donor insemination from a cross-cultural perspective, as social scientists contribute accounts and analyses of assisted conception around the world.

Gosden, Roger. *Designing Babies: The Brave New World of Reproductive Technology*. W. H. Freeman, 2000. This literary and philosophical work explores medical history as well as current developments in reproductive technology. The author has worked with Robert Edwards, who was responsible for the first "test-tube" baby (Louise Brown, conceived through IVF).

Humes, Edward. *Baby E.R.: The Heroic Doctors and Nurses Who Perform Medicine's Tiniest Miracles*. New York: Simon & Schuster, 2000. Edward Humes was inspired to write this account of advanced technologies for treating newborns when his own daughter spent a week in the emergency room with a severe kidney infection. Humes's account of the treatments available to premature babies makes it clear that the age of viability—when a child can exist outside the womb—is getting earlier and earlier. He also eloquently describes the medical problems attendant on multiple births, which are often premature and result in babies with low birth weights.

Kearney, Brian. *High-Tech Conception: A Comprehensive Handbook for Consumers*. New York: Bantam Books, 1998. The author argues that numerous risks accompany high-tech fertility treatments.

Kimbrell, Andrew. *The Human Body Shop: The Cloning, Engineering, and Marketing of Life*. Washington, D.C.: Regnery Publishing, 1998. Featuring an introduction by Bernard Nathanson, known as a bitter opponent of abortion, and a foreword by Jeremy Rifkin, a left-wing opponent of biotechnology, Kimbrell's work calls for ending the buying and selling of the human body, in the form of blood donations, organ transplants, artificial insemination, and surrogate motherhood, arguing that the poor will always be exploited by the rich if such transactions are permitted. Kimbrell is the policy director of the Foundation on Economic Trends, headed by Jeremy Rifkin.

168

Annotated Bibliography

Kolata, Gina Bari. *Clone: The Road to Dolly and the Path Ahead.* New York: William Morrow, 1999. The *New York Times* science reporter gives a full account of the development of Dolly, the sheep cloned by Scottish livestock scientists in 1997; she also covers the century-old history of cloning, and the social conflicts that have accompanied this controversial research.

Lublin, Nancy. *Pandora's Box: Feminism Confronts Reproductive Technology.* Lanham, Md.: Rowman & Littlefield, 1998. An exploration of the various ways that feminists have responded to advances in reproductive technology, from technophilia (love of technology) to technophobia (fear of technology), concluding with a call for praxis feminism, combining theoretical insights with practical experience.

Marrs, Richard, M.D., with Lisa Friedman Bloch and Kathy Kirtland Silverman. *Dr. Richard Marrs' Fertility Book: America's Leading Infertility Expert Tells You Everything You Need to Know About Getting Pregnant.* New York: Dell, 1998. Marrs, the fertility specialist who in 1985 achieved the first birth in the United States from a frozen embryo, reviews the panoply of reproductive technology options available when his book came out in 1998.

McCuen, Gary E., ed. *Cloning: Science and Society (Ideas in Conflict Series).* Hudson, Wis.: Gem Publications, 1998. A series of essays geared especially for high school and college-age readers, giving an overview of the cloning issue and the various responses to it.

Merrick, Janna C., and Robert H. Blank, eds. *The Politics of Pregnancy: Policy Dilemmas in the Maternal-Fetal Relationship.* New York: Haworth, 1994. A collection of essays on policy issues that relate to the relationship between pregnant woman and fetus, analyzing such topics as reproductive technology, surrogate motherhood, in utero experimentation, court-ordered obstetrical interventions, neonatal drug testing, workplace hazards for pregnant women, and abortion. Although published several years ago, this volume still offers a useful perspective on current issues.

Meyer, Cheryl L. *The Wandering Uterus: Politics and the Reproductive Rights of Women.* New York: NYU Press, 1997. A look at the way in which society's ideas about female sexuality affect the practice of law and medicine, in light of advances in reproductive technology.

Pence, Gregory E. *Who's Afraid of Human Cloning?* Lanham, Md.: Rowman & Littlefield, 1998. Pence, a medical ethicist and philosopher, is supportive of cloning and critical of those who would disseminate horror stories about it. He asserts that many arguments against cloning were previously used against IVF, which is now widely accepted. He also argues that women need to be included in the debate over cloning.

Pence, Gregory E., ed. *Flesh of My Flesh: The Ethics of Cloning Humans: A Reader.* Lanham, Md.: Rowman & Littlefield, 1998. A collection of 13 essays representing a variety of scientific perspectives on cloning, written in response to the 1997 cloning of Dolly, the sheep (except for a 1971 article by James Watson, winner of the Nobel Prize for discovering DNA and first head of the Human Genome Project). Contributors to the book include Stephen Jay Gould and the National Bioethics Advisory Commission.

Raymond, Janice. *Women as Wombs*. San Francisco: HarperCollins, 1993. The author argues that women are pressured to fulfill childbearing roles, not just in the United States but around the world.

Silber, Sherman J. *How to Get Pregnant: With the New Technology*. New York: Warner Books, 1998. A doctor explains fertility treatments, offering readable, accessible explanations of the latest fertility technologies as of 1998. Silber is extremely enthusiastic about reproductive technology, which he argues should be covered by medical insurance, since, he claims, infertility can lead to increased risk of ovarian, breast, and uterine cancer in older women.

Silver, Lee M. *Remaking Eden: How Genetic Engineering and Cloning Will Transform the American Family*. New York: Avon, 1998. Silver's view on genetic engineering is one of cautious optimism. He explains the range of ways that new reproductive technologies might remake human families and lives.

Squier, Susan Merrill. *Babies in Bottles: Twentieth-Century Visions of Reproductive Technology*. New Brunswick, N.J.: Rutgers University Press, 1994. The author looks at early-twentieth-century fiction and popular science writing to get a perspective on contemporary reproductive technology and our relationship to it.

Wilmut, Ian, Keith Campbell, and Colin Tudge. *The Second Creation: Dolly and the Age of Biological Control*. New York: Farrar, Straus & Giroux, 2000. An account by Wilmut and Campbell, the Scottish researchers who created the first successful clone of a sheep in 1997, working with veteran science writer Tudge. The authors explain the basic biology involved in cloning and help distinguish facts from myths.

ARTICLES

REPRODUCTIVE RIGHTS

Newspapers and Magazines

Abel, David. "Jailed Mother Gets Unsolicited Help." *Boston Globe*. September 2, 2000, p. B.1. Rebecca Corneau, suspected of neglect in the death of her last baby, is jailed while pregnant because she refuses medical help and prenatal exams on religious grounds; women's groups come to her defense.

————. "RU-486 Access Divides College Campuses." *Boston Globe*. January 27, 2001, p. A.1. Colleges and universities are not sure how to respond to RU-486 for fear of alienating donors; so far Yale University is the only college to have publicly promised to provide the drug.

Allina, Amy. "Early Abortion Drug: Science Prevails . . . At Last!" *Network News*. January/February 2001, 26:1, p. 5. Despite political opposition, science has finally prevailed in the matter of RU-486; a pro-choice article in the National Women's Health Network publication.

"American Life League: In Defense of Women's Rights . . . and the Real State of World Population 2000; Press Conference and Protest of UNFPA's Annual State of World Population Report." *PR Newswire*. September 19, 2000, p. 1. The American Life League (ALL) predicts "imminent world population collapse" and wants to save poor indigenous women throughout the world from the UN Population Fund's "anti-Christian population elimination agenda," which, the ALL claims, it advocates under a deceptive "banner of reproductive rights, AIDS prevention, gender equality and sexual rights."

"American Life League: In-Vitro Fertilization Caters to Couples Who Prefer Abortion Under Glass." *PR Newswire*. February 7, 2001, p. 1. Father Joseph Howard, executive director of the American Bioethics Advisory Commission (a division of the American Life League), argues that "Fertility treatments which destroy human beings do not constitute basic human rights and should in no way be covered by health insurance."

Arkes, Hadley. "On the Born-Alive Infants Protection Act of 2000." *Human Life Review*. Fall 2000, 26:4, p. 15. A transcript of the author's testimony before Congress on HR-4292, the "Born-Alive Infants Protection Act," published in a pro-life journal.

Armas, Genaro C. "Women Inching Closer to Equality, Report Says." (Albany) *Times Union*. November 16, 2000, p. A.8. According to a report from the Institute for Women's Policy Research, gains in education and income and an increased political presence have helped women improve their social and economic status—yet women are still far from achieving equality with men. The Institute ranks each state on women's rights, including reproductive rights.

Arthur, Joyce. "No, Virginia, Abortion Is Not Genocide." *The Humanist*. July/August 2000, 60:4, p. 20. A passionate critique of the Center for Bio-Ethical Reform's portrayal of abortion as comparable to the Holocaust and the lynching of African Americans, published in the journal of the American Humanist Association.

"Ashcroft Is Only Part of a Bush Abortion Backlash." *San Francisco Chronicle.* January 18, 2001, p. A. 24. An editorial indicating that John Ashcroft will roll back protections of a woman's right to choose.

Baumgardner, Jennifer. "The Missing Link." *Ms.* December 2000/January 2001, 11:1, p. 19. A look at *Mattson v. Red River Women's Clinic,* in which a pro-life activist is trying to prevent an abortion clinic from stating that medical research does not show that abortion causes breast cancer.

Belluck, Pam. "After Abortion Victory, Doctor's Troubles Persist." *New York Times.* November 7, 2000, p. A. 18. A look at the difficulties faced by Dr. Leroy Carhart, the doctor involved in *Stenberg v. Carhart,* the 2000 Supreme Court case on "partial-birth" abortion. Despite the fact that Carhart won the suit, he has faced harassment and professional penalties as a result of his pro-choice stance.

"Bishops and the Politicians: A Bad Mix." *National Catholic Reporter.* August 11, 2000, 36:36, p. 28. Bishops must now blame themselves for inappropriate involvement in the presidential election around the issue of abortion.

"Bitter Pills." *Christianity Today.* December 4, 2000, 44:14, p. 31. A discussion of the controversy over RU-486, arguing that pro-life Americans must work within a culture that treats pregnancy as a disease and abortion as the cure.

"Blacks Are Killing the Race, Say Advocates." *Michigan Chronicle.* July 12, 2000, p. B.4. The National Black Pro-Life Congress held its third annual Celebration of Life Conference in Michigan, with Reggie White and Alveda King-Tookes, Martin Luther King's niece, as speakers.

Blunt, Sheryl Henderson. "Pushing Bush Right." *Christianity Today.* March 5, 2001, 45:4, p. 84. Blunt discusses lobbying efforts that might push Bush to the right on pro-life matters, religious freedom, and faith-based initiatives.

Bouchard, Charles E. "How Could a Catholic Vote That Way." *America.* 184:4, p. 12. A look at the Catholic support for Al Gore in the 2000 election, despite Gore's support for abortion rights.

Branch-Brioso, Karen. "Bush Gives Anti-Abortion Cause New Life; New President Tells Activists: 'We Share a Great Goal': Protesters March in D.C. on Roe v. Wade Anniversary." *St. Louis Post-Dispatch.* January 23, 2001, p. A.1. Coverage of pro-choice and pro-life activity in Washington on the anniversary of *Roe v. Wade* and the election of a pro-life president.

Byrne, Harry J. "A Pro-Life Strategy of Persuasion." *America.* January 22–January 29, 2001, 184:2, p. 12. An argument for pro-lifers to affirm the legitimate liberty and equality of women as a way to be more effective politically.

Casey, Laurie. "A Reality Check on Abortion; Activists Point Out Some Myths and Gray Areas in Reproductive Rights; Reality." *Chicago Tribune.* January 31, 2001, p. 3. A report on a pro-choice meeting featuring a range of people: a pro-choice high school senior; a female pastor of a pro-choice church; people from activist groups; and a disability-rights activist.

Chinni, Dante. "Parsing Bush's Mixed Messages on Abortion; Recent Steps Reflect Antiabortion Stand, But Some Say Bush's Actions Will Be Limited." *Christian Science Monitor.* January 25, 2001, p. 2. Despite President Bush's apparently moderate stance, Bush has opened the abortion debate in a contentious way by nominating John Ashcroft attorney general.

Claiborne, William. "Abortion Foes Want States to Curb RU-486." *Washington Post.* October 5, 2000, p. A.1. Legislative directors or heads of nearly two dozen antiabortion groups in some of the most antiabortion states say that they are looking to include RU-486 in current laws that restrict access to abortion, including parental consent laws, waiting periods for abortions, and bans on public funding for abortions or abortion-related counseling.

Copeland, Libby. "For an Abortion Opponent, RU-486 Is a Bitter Pill." *Washington Post.* September 30, 2000, p. C.1. A portrait of pro-life activist Mary Ann Kreitzer's sorrow over the decision to legalize RU-486.

Crossette, Barbara. "Working for Women's Sexual Rights." *New York Times.* October 2, 2000, p. A.8. A profile of Dr. Nafis Sadik, a 71-year-old Muslim from India who has spent her life working for women's sexual rights.

Dao, James. "Ringing Phones, Chiming Doorbells, Stuffed E-Mailboxes: The Great Voter Roundup." *New York Times.* November 7, 2000, p. A.22. A look at the way pro-choice activists mobilized to try to elect Al Gore.

DeMarco, Donald. "The Reality of Motherhood." *Human Life Review.* Fall 2000, 26:4, p. 47. The author argues that by having an abortion, a woman abandons her spiritual relationship with motherhood, causing pregnancy to be viewed as an invasion rather than as a uniting mother-child relationship.

Donovan, Gill. "Pro-Life Leader Decries 'Pro-Abortion McCarthyism'." *National Catholic Reporter.* January 26, 2001, 37:13, p. 8. The U.S. bishops' pro-life spokeswoman accuses the opponents of Bush's cabinet nominees of "proabortion McCarthyism."

Dowling, Katherine. "Prolife Doctors Should Have Choices, Too." *U.S. Catholic.* March 2001, 66:3, p. 24. The author of this article, a doctor, worries that medicine is being transformed from a healing profession into a form of social engineering.

Eastlick, Megan. "Australia: Fertility Services for Single Women." *Off Our Backs.* October 2000, 30:9, p. 3. A federal court rules that the Australian state of Victoria can no longer prohibit single women—including lesbians—from receiving state-funded fertility services.

Estrich, Susan. "For Some, Choice Gets Harder." *Nation.* October 9, 2000, 271:10, p. 19. Estrich analyzes the threat posed to reproductive rights by the Supreme Court: She does not believe that abortion will be rendered illegal, that doctors will be locked up for providing abortions, or that middle-class women will have difficulty terminating early-stage pregnancies; but she does foresee severe restrictions on a woman's right to choose, and she argues that poor women or women in rural areas already have difficulty obtaining access to abortion.

Feldt, Gloria. "Keep Choice in Mind." *New York Times.* December 26, 2000, p. A.31. The author, president of the Planned Parenthood Federation of America, expresses her concern about what she views as President George W. Bush's disregard of reproductive rights.

Fenoglio, Gia, and Erin Heath. "Another Front in the Abortion Wars." *National Journal.* February 10, 2001, 33:6, p. 432. Abortion rights opponents say that parental notification laws can be effective in reducing abortions.

Fishman, Steve. "Body Politics." *Harper's Bazaar.* September 2000, Issue 3455, p. 520. A discussion of the various ways that abortion has been restricted and limited, which complicates the pro-life vs. pro-choice issue.

Foreman, Judy. "The Time Has Dawned for 'Morning-After' Contraception." *Boston Globe.* January 30, 2001. The author, a health columnist, points out that emergency or "morning-after" contraception should be widely and easily available, an idea that even the American Medical Association supports. The National Right to Life Committee has not opposed this type of contraception.

Fowler, Anne, Nicki Nichols Gamble, Frances X. Hogan, Melissa Kogut, Madeline McComish, and Barbara Thorp. "Talking with the Enemy for Nearly Six Years, Leaders on Both Sides of the Abortion Debate Have Met in Secret in an Attempt to Better Understand Each Other, Now They Are Ready to Share What They Have Learned." *Boston Globe.* January 28, 2001, p. F.1. In response to John Salvi's 20-minute shooting spree at two abortion clinics in 1994, pro-choice and pro-life advocates came together to try to resolve the bitter divisions between the two movements; this article reports on their encounters.

"FRC and Pro-Life Coalition Send Pro-Life Message to Democratic Convention, Launch TV Ad Campaign in Los Angeles." *PR Newswire.* August 14, 2000, p. 1. A coalition of pro-life groups, including Family Research Council (FRC), launches a TV ad campaign called "Second Thoughts About Abortion."

"'Gag Rule' Keeps Aid from the Needy." *Atlanta Constitution.* July 19, 2000, p. A.18. An editorial opposing the "gag rule," which bars mention of abortion by international family planning associations.

Garvey, Megan. "Convention 2000/The Democratic Convention: Abortion Foes Choose Life Within the Party; A Small Faction of Democrats Soldiers on With a Message More at Home in the GOP. But the Dissidents Say They're Not Moving From Their Position, or Their Political Base."

Los Angeles Times. August 17, 2000, p. U.3. Antiabortion Democrats say that their party does not welcome them and will not let them speak.

Gibbs, Nancy. "The Pill Arrives." *Time.* October 9, 2000, 156:15, p. 40. Abortion rates in the United States have been declining, but pro-life advocates are worried about the effect of the "abortion pill," RU-486.

Glaberson, William. "Foes of Abortion Start New Effort After Court Loss." *New York Times.* June 30, 2000, p. A.1. A day after *Stenberg v. Carhart* strikes down the Nebraska law banning "partial-birth abortion," supporters of the ban are planning more laws to restrict abortion procedures.

"Global Gag Rule Backfires." *Denver Post.* January 24, 2001, p. B.08. An editorial pointing out that family planning agencies that come under the gag rule also promote birth control so that women can avoid abortions; if women seek illegal abortions, says the editorial, these groups must be able to counsel them, or the women will die.

Goldkamp, Richard J. "The Scheidler Case: Conning the Court with RICO." *Human Life Review.* Fall 2000, 26:4, p. 27. NOW was suing Joseph Scheidler, leader of several abortion clinic protests, using the RICO laws as their basis; Goldkamp feels that NOW has manipulated jurors' views of the pro-life movement.

Goodman, Ellen. "Bush's Attack on the Poorest Women." *Boston Globe.* January 25, 2001, p. A.13. Goodman points out that under the gag rule that Bush has imposed in international family planning clinics, a woman is not allowed to hear about abortion as an option, even if is legal in her country.

———. "Is It True? Is the Strife About Abortion Over?" *Boston Globe.* October 1, 2000, p. E.7. The columnist celebrates the FDA approval of RU-486 and wonders how the pro-life movement will respond. She is concerned for the future of the abortion debate.

Guzy, M.W. "From Dolly to Dilemma." *St. Louis Post-Dispatch.* January 31, 2000, p. B.7. A look at British law on cloning and on the legal and ethical conflicts that cloning raises.

Hansen, Ronald J. "Plan Pays Addicts to Be Sterilized; Women Offered $200 in Effort to Stop Drug-Dependent Births." *Detroit News.* December 8, 2000, p. 07. An account of a plan that pays drug-addicted women to be sterilized.

Hines, Cragg. "Ashcroft Falters as Quick-Change Artist." *Houston Chronicle.* January 18, 2001, p. 24. A report from the midst of the confirmation hearings on Attorney General nominee John Ashcroft, pointing out the contradictions between Ashcroft's lifelong conservative positions on abortion and other issues and his claims to the Senate that he would uphold the laws he had spent his life trying to change.

Howard, Trisha L. "Arms of Love Hopes New Equipment Will Assist in Fight to Stop Abortions; Pregnant Women Can View Ultrasound." *St.*

Louis Post-Dispatch. September 7, 2000, p. SM.1. The Arms of Love Pregnancy Resource Center make ultrasound available to pregnant women in the hopes that seeing their babies' images will keep the women from choosing abortion.

Kaufman, Marc. "Abortion Pill Deliveries Begin Soon; Long-Delayed RU-486 to Be Available Within Days at Doctors' Offices, Clinics." *Washington Post*. November 16, 2000, p. A.2. Despite the FDA approval of RU-486, the battle is not over, as doctors must now be persuaded to prescribe the pill.

Kendall, Mary Claire. "More Than One Choice." *American Enterprise*. October/November 2000, 11:7, p.14. Feminists for Life is a group that tries to show college women that a pro-choice stance does not really affirm womanhood.

Kleiman, Carol. "Flexible Workplace Makes Honesty the Best Policy." *Chicago Tribune*. January 9, 2001, p. 1. A look at how employees undergoing fertility treatment handle workplace issues.

Kornblut, Anne E. "Bush Taps Ashcroft for Attorney General." *Boston Globe*. December 23, 2000, p. A.1. A report on President George W. Bush's nomination of Missouri senator John Ashcroft, a deeply religious Christian who opposes abortion rights but who nevertheless asserts his intention to uphold existing laws.

Krauthammer, Charles. "Why Pro-Lifers Are Missing the Point." *Time*. February 12, 2001, 157:6, p.60. An article supporting stem-cell research and criticizing the pro-life movement for opposing it.

Kuttner, Robert. "For Many Voters, A Choice About Choice." *Boston Globe*. October 15, 2000, p. C.7. Despite the historically pro-life positions of Republicans George W. Bush and Dick Cheney, their presidential campaign has sounded "kinder and gentler" on abortion rights. Kuttner, co-editor of the conservative magazine *The American Prospect*, attributes their position to the "phenomenally successful organizing campaign" mounted by reproductive rights groups such as NARAL and Planned Parenthood.

Lace, Candi. "Abortion and Obscenity: Anti-Choice Group Makes Hideous Connections." *Off Our Backs*. January 2001, 31:1, p. 5. An article criticizing the Center for Bio-Ethical Reform's "Genocide Awareness Project," which compares abortion to historical examples of genocide.

Leonard, Mary. "New Tactics Shift Sentiments on Abortion." *Boston Globe*. July 16, 2000, p. E.1. Although the Supreme Court ruled against right-to-lifers in *Stenberg v. Carhart*, their larger strategy is working: to restrict abortion and shift public sentiment against it.

———. "Ruling Galvanizes Antiabortion Forces to Press on for Ban." *Boston Globe*. June 30, 2000, p. A.3. In response to their loss in *Stenberg v.*

Carhart, antiabortion activists are energized to demand that Bush give abortion a more central place in his campaign.

Lerner, Sharon. "Reading Between the Lines." *Village Voice*, February 6, 2001, 46:5, p. 56. The author discusses Ashcroft's possible attempts to overturn *Roe v. Wade*.

Lochhead, Carolyn. "Abortion Policy Reversed/Bush Bans Use of Federal Funds for Overseas Abortion Counseling." *San Francisco Chronicle*. January 23, 2001, p. A.1. Anti-abortion demonstrators protested the anniversary of *Roe v. Wade*, as Bush institutes the gag rule on mention of abortion at international family planning clinics.

Lombardi, Kate Stone. "A Clinic Where All the Doctors Are Women." *New York Times*. December 3, 2000, p, 14WC.8. A clinic offers a full range of ob/gyn services by nine women doctors at Montefiore Larchmont Women's Center, in the New York City suburb of Larchmont.

Lueck, Sarah. "Abortion Foes Face Tough Battle Against RU-486 Drug." *Wall Street Journal*. February 12, 2001, p. A.28. Antiabortion activists will have trouble getting the "abortion pill" outlawed, even with abortion foe Tommy Thompson at the head of the Department of Health and Human Services.

Luna, Christopher. "Kate Michelman." *Current Biography*. November 2000, 61:11, p. 64. A profile of Kate Michelman, founder and president of the National Abortion and Reproductive Rights Action League (NARAL), describing how Michelman has brought the group from a small grassroots organization into a major political voice.

Malcolm, Teresa. "Abortion Foes Decry Stabbing of Doctor." *National Catholic Reporter*. July 28, 2000, 36:35, p. 12. Canadian bishops condemn the stabbing of an abortion provider in Vancouver.

———. "Congress Defends Vatican UN Status." *National Catholic Reporter*. July 28, 2000, 36:35, p. 10. Catholics for a Free Choice, a Catholic group whose pro-choice position puts them at odds with the Vatican, has spearheaded a "See Change Campaign" to strip the Vatican of its permanent observer status, which allows Vatican diplomats to speak in debates and participate in UN conferences. The Vatican hails a congressional resolution defending the Vatican's observer status.

———. "Priests for Life Launch Campaign for Election Year." *National Catholic Reporter*. July 28, 2000, 36:35, p. 11. Priests for Life wants voters to remember the importance of abortion in an election year.

Mann, Judy. "Mobilizing the Family Planning Vote." *Washington Post*. October 11, 2000, p. C.13. A national survey commissioned by Planned Parenthood has found that half to two-thirds of those surveyed said that certain reproductive rights issues were important enough to influence their votes. Planned Parenthood head Gloria Feldt discusses the issues and explores their significance for the coming presidential election.

———. "Reduce Abortion and Disarm the Far Right." *Washington Post.* December 1, 2000, p. C.11. As abortions become less necessary, more private, and more available, pro-life activists will have less ammunition for their cause.

Marinucci, Carla. "Nader and Bush Agree on Fate of *Roe vs. Wade*/Both Say 1973 Decision Won't Be Overturned Under Next President." *San Francisco Chronicle.* November 4, 2000, p. A.4. Both Green Party candidate Ralph Nader and GOP candidate George W. Bush agree that if Bush is elected, it will not affect the Supreme Court's 1973 *Roe v. Wade* decision upholding a woman's right to an abortion. Although both men agree that the next president will have enormous influence on reproductive rights, they also assert that *Roe v. Wade* will not be overturned.

McCombs, Brady. "Vote Outcome Splits Anti-Abortion Groups." *Denver Post.* November 12, 2000, p. B.02. Colorado Right to Life opposes Amendment 25—a mandatory 24-hour waiting period before getting an abortion.

McGinley, Laurie. "HHS Choice Upsets Antiabortion Allies Over Stem Cells." *Wall Street Journal.* January 16, 2001, p. A.28. Antiabortion groups are not sure about Tommy Thompson's credentials as the Wisconsin governor is nominated to head the Department of Health and Human Services.

McKibben, Ginny. "Abortion Foes Fight Arapahoe Picket Line." *Denver Post.* January 16, 2001, p. B.02. Abortion protestors are battling a new county law banning pickets at the homes of doctors who provide abortions.

McNelly, Dave. "The Democratic Convention: Abortion Highlighted as Issue to Show Differences with GOP." *Atlanta Constitution.* August 18, 2000, p. B.4. The National Abortion and Reproductive Rights Action League (NARAL) is actively working to remind delegates to the Democratic Convention in Atlanta that choice is a crucial issue for the coming election—and the GOP candidates have a long history of opposing reproductive rights.

Mehren, Elizabeth. "Pregnant Sect Member's Case Is a Rights Quandary; Religion; Fears for Kids in the Group that Uses Prayer Instead of Medicine Prompts a Confinement Order." *Los Angeles Times.* September 9, 2000, p. 1. Rebecca Corneau has been placed in protective custody while pregnant to protect the unborn child, as she is committed to refusing medical assistance for religious reasons and is suspected in the death of her infant son. Feminist groups are outraged at what they see as the infringement of Corneau's rights, and the dangerous precedent the court's ruling sets for other pregnant women.

Miller, John J. "What Now, Lifers?" *National Review.* February 19, 2001, 53:3, p. 22. The pro-life movement should stop trying to ban "partial-birth abortions," argues the author, since any woman who wants such a procedure can almost certainly get an abortion another way.

Mitchell, Alison. "Senate Confirms Ashcroft as Attorney General, 58–42, Closing a Five-Week Battle." *New York Times.* February 2, 2001, p. A.1. The Senate confirms Missouri senator John Ashcroft as attorney general in a 58–42 vote, even though some Senate Democrats objected to Ashcroft in part because of his long record of pro-life activities.

Moore, Julianne. "Abortion Rights—You Could Lose Yours." *Glamour.* July 2000, 98:7, p. 113. Actress Julianne Moore encourages women to express their opinions on reproductive rights by voting, since, she says, just a few pieces of legislation could eradicate those rights. Moore points out that since 1994, Congress has voted nearly 140 times to restrict reproductive rights.

Morrison, Jacqueline. "Is Approval of Abortion Pill Welcome? YES: RU-486 Helps Reproductive Rights With Safe, Early Option for Abortion." *Detroit News.* October 10, 2000, p. 9. The author, head of Planned Parenthood of Southeast Michigan, argues that antiabortion forces have marginalized abortion into a procedure performed by only a few doctors in easily identifiable clinics. She asserts that RU-486, the "abortion pill," will make it easier for women to have access to abortion while they and their doctors protect their privacy.

Morrison, Patt. "A President Rowing in Reverse on Abortion Issues." *Los Angeles Times.* January 26, 2001, p. B.1. A look at what the new president will do about abortion.

Murphy, Shelley. "Court Gives Go-Ahead on Buffer Zones; State to Enforce Its New Law for Abortion Clinics." *Boston Globe.* December 23, 2000, p. A.1. A federal appeals court has lifted a ban on enforcing "buffer zones" around abortion clinics—zones that antiabortion protestors are not allowed to cross.

Oliphant, Thomas. "Abortion Politics." *Boston Globe.* July 4, 2000, p. A.11. "Partial-birth abortion" will no longer be the central issue; now abortion itself will be at stake.

"Partial Rebirth." *Washington Post.* July 3, 2000, p. A.18. An editorial supporting the Supreme Court's action in *Stenberg v. Carhart.*

Paulson, Michael. "Fetus Dispute Brings Wider Issues to Fore." *Boston Globe.* September 10, 2000, p. B.5. A discussion of the Rebecca Corneau case, in which the state has taken a pregnant woman into custody to protect her unborn child from the woman's failure to obtain medical care.

Pearson, Patricia. "Abortion Fringes Drown Out Voices from Vast Middle." *USA Today.* January 31, 2001, p. A.15. The author argues that both pro- and antiabortion activists are taking hard-line positions out of touch with the majority of the American people, and calls for more complex and nuanced positions on abortion, which the author believes will more accurately reflect the views of most U.S. citizens.

"Placating Abortion Foes." *Boston Globe.* January 24, 2001, p. A.14. An editorial criticizing Bush's institution of a global gag rule.

Pollitt, Katha. "Antichoice Intimidation." *Nation.* December 11, 2000, 271:19, p. 6. The feminist columnist discusses how clinics and providers are falling victim to an increasing number of attacks in the local courts.

"The Privacy Pill." *St. Louis Post-Dispatch.* September 29, 2000, p. C.14. An editorial asserting that the FDA approval of RU-486 "is likely to rekindle rather than resolve our national debate on abortion."

Rein, Lisa, and Craig Timberg. "Abortion Bill Gains in Senate; Panel Passes 1-Day Wait; House Backs Contraception Measure." *Washington Post.* February 1, 2001, p. B.7. The Virginia House of Representatives gives preliminary approval to a law that would allow pharmacists to distribute a "morning-after pill" without a doctor's prescription; meanwhile, the Virginia Senate considers informed consent legislation that would require a woman seeking an abortion to wait 24 hours beefore receiving it.

Rein, Lisa, and William Branigin. "Virginia Approves Limits on Abortion; Assembly Conservatives Affirm 24-hour Delay." *Washington Post.* February 7, 2001, p. A 1. Informed consent legislation, requiring a mandatory waiting period and the mandatory viewing of pictures of fetal development before a woman can obtain an abortion, cleared the Virginia General Assembly; this is considered a major milestone for conservatives seeking to restrict women's access to abortion. The article interviews a range of politicians, abortion providers, and activists on their response to the bill.

Roiphe, Katie. "Women: Back to the Back Alley: Last Monday Was George Bush's First Day in Office. It Also Just Happened to Be the 28th Anniversary of the Supreme Court Ruling That Gave American Women the Right to Abortion. Katie Roiphe Reports from New York on How the President Marked the Day." *The Guardian.* January 29, 2001, p. 2.11. The columnist looks at the election of a pro-life president and calls for renewed commitment to choice.

Rosin, Hanna. "Decision Forces Foes to Revamp Strategy." *Washington Post.* September 29, 2000, p. A.1. The acceptance of RU-486 will require pro-life activists to come up with new political strategies.

Roth, Bennett. "Bush Halts Funding Used for Abortions." *Houston Chronicle.* January 23, 2001, p. A.1. Bush's executive order on abortion mirrors the policies of the Reagan and Bush administrations.

Annotated Bibliography

"RU-486." *America*. October 14, 2000, 183:11, p. 3. Pro-life supporters suffered a defeat when RU-486 was approved.

Salladay, Robert. "New Wind in Their Sails/Abortion Protesters in D.C. Applaud Bush's Move but Want National Change." *San Francisco Chronicle*. January 23, 2001, p. A.6. Abortion protestors are concerned about Bush's appointments to the Supreme Court.

Schmich, Mary. "RU-486 Side Effect Is Making Abortion Key Election Issue." *Chicago Tribune*. October 1, 2000, p. 4C.1. A look at the impact of RU-486 on the presidential election.

Schoettler, Gail. "'Right to Know' Is Wrong." *Denver Post*. October 29, 2000, p. M2. A column criticizing the "right-to-know" provision, Amendment 25, that will go before the Colorado electorate. The author argues that the law's intent is not to inform women but to restrict abortion.

Sevcik, Kim. "The Baby Abandonment Myth." *Ms.* October/November 2000, 10:6, p. 34. The author argues that the right-to-life movement has been involved in legislation to decriminalize "safe surrender," in which women can leave their newborns with emergency medical technicians.

Simon, Stephanie. "Small-Town Doctors Weigh Principle, Pressure and Abortion Pill." *Los Angeles Times*. November 21, 2000, p. A.1. A look at RU-486 and how people in Rapid City, South Dakota, are responding to it.

"Stenberg v. Carhart." *Human Life Review*. Fall 2000, 26:4, p. 86. A pro-life analysis of the Supreme Court decision.

Stockman, Farah. "Pregnant Woman in Bid to Reverse Attleboro Ruling." *Boston Globe*. September 6, 2000, p. B.2. Feminist lawyer Wendy Murphy argues against a court decision placing pregnant woman Rebecca Corneau into protective custody to prevent her unborn child from the consequences of Corneau's refusal on religious grounds to accept medical assistance. Murphy cites another pregnant client's interest, asking, "What if my client rides a unicycle, climbs a ladder, or skydives during pregnancy? Is someone going to take her into custody?"

Swift, Pat. "A Call to Action for Supporters of Abortion Rights." *Buffalo News*. July 8, 2000, p. C.9. Despite the recent Supreme Court pro-choice ruling, *Stenberg v. Carhart*, abortion rights activists continue to be concerned about increasing restrictions on women's reproductive choice. The article covers the views of *Nation* columnist Katha Pollitt and New York lawyer Cynthia L. Cooper, prominent pro-choice feminists.

Terry, Sara. "Whose Family? The Revolt of the Child-Free." *Christian Science Monitor*. August 29, 2000, p. 1. A look at the conflicts between people who have children and people who choose not to.

Thompson, Ginger. "A Victory of Sorts for Abortion Rights in a Mexican State." *New York Times*. August 29, 2000, p. A.3. Abortion rights groups

in Mexico welcome the decision of a conservative governor of Guanaju-
ato to effectively veto a bill that would have extended a ban on abortions
to cases of rape.

Toner, Robin. "Bush Caught in the Middle on Research on Stem Cells."
New York Times. February 18, 2001, p. 1.18. An exploration of the stem
cell debate.

———. "Opponents of Abortions Cheer New Administration." *New York
Times.* January 23, 2001, p. A.16. A look at the antiabortion stance of the
Bush administration.

———. "A Tactical Challenge." *New York Times.* September 30, 2000,
p. A.10. An exploration of the ways that both the pro-choice and pro-life
movements have changed tactics over the years.

"A Victory for Choice." *Buffalo News.* September 30, 2000, p. B6. An editorial that argues that FDA approval of RU-486 is welcome, but will not result in the flood of abortions that pro-life groups have predicted.

"Vote Anti-Abortion in Upcoming Election, Catholic Leaders Urge."
Church & State. November 2000, 53:10, p. 16. The Roman Catholic hi-
erarchy seems to be becoming more active in electoral politics.

Wallace, Alicia. "FDA Approval of Mifepristone Immediately Targeted."
National NOW Times, Winter 2001, 32:4, p. 2. NOW responds enthusiastically to the FDA's September 29th approval of RU-486; however,
NOW is concerned that opponents of reproductive choice will seek to restrict access to the medication.

Weiss, Rick. "Thompson Signals He'll Initiate New HHS Review of Abortion Drug." *Washington Post.* January 20, 2001, p. A.8. Longtime abortion
foe Wisconsin governor Tommy G. Thompson is appointed head of Department of Health and Human Services by President-elect George W.
Bush; Thompson hints that he will review the FDA's approval of RU-486.

Will, George F. "An Act of Judicial Infamy." *Human Life Review.* Fall 2000,
26:4, p. 133. The conservative columnist opposes *Stenberg v. Carhart*, the
2000 Supreme Court decision overturning a ban on "partial-birth abortion."

———. "The Partial-Birth Censors." *Washington Post.* August 20, 2000,
p. B.7. The conservative columnist criticizes a *Post* decision not to publish a pro-life ad on "partial-birth" abortion.

Wingert, Pat. "The Next Abortion Battle." *Newsweek.* July 10, 2000, 136:2,
p. 24. A look at the ways that Leroy Carhart, the doctor involved in *Stenberg v. Carhart*, has been harassed for his pro-choice activities.

"Women and Health." *WIN News.* Summer 2000, 26:3, p. 22. An overview
of several women's health issues, claiming that "anthropologists who observe professional midwives . . . increasingly note that . . . professional
midwives often treat women very badly during birth, ignoring their needs
and requests."

Annotated Bibliography

"World Youth Alliance: UNICEF Causes Scandal With Halloween Boxes." *PR Newswire.* October 26, 2000, p. 1. The World Youth Alliance, a pro-life group, accuses UNICEF of actively promoting abortion and sexual rights to children.

Zagaroli, Lisa. "Partial-birth Ruling Sets Abortion Battle Lines; Right to Life Says It Will Push State Courts to Define When Procedure Becomes Infanticide." *Detroit News.* June 30, 2000, p. A.1. A look at the political fallout from the Supreme Court decision, *Stenberg v. Carhart.*

Zimmerman, Rachel. "Wrangling Over Abortion Intensifies as RU-486 Pill Nears the Market." *Wall Street Journal.* November 14, 2000, p. B.1. As Danco Laboratories LLC sets a high price for RU-486, activists demand a price that will make the medication more accessible.

Zorn, Eric. "Abortion Debate Unlikely to Find Middle Ground." *Chicago Tribune.* February 13, 2001, p. 2C.1. A look at the difficulties of bringing pro-choice and pro-life forces together.

Specialized Journals

Brown, Robert W. "Provider Availability, Race, and Abortion Demand." *Southern Economic Journal.* January 2001, 67:3, p. 656. Variations in the extent to which abortion is available may affect the demand for abortion, argues this article, pointing out that travel costs to far-off abortion providers add greatly to the cost of an abortion and thereby affect a person's tendency to choose the procedure.

Gennaro, Rocco J. "A Note on Abortion and Capital Punishment." *International Philosophy Quarterly.* December 2000, 40:4, p. 491. A discussion of how anti-capital punishment arguments can be used against abortion, and vice versa.

Glynn, Judith. "Decreased Fertility Among HIV-1-infected Women Attending Antenatal Clinics in Three African Cities." *Journal of Acquired Immune Deficiency Syndromes.* December 1, 2000, 25:4, p. 345. An exploration of conditions affecting the fertility of HIV-infected African women.

Mason, Karen Oppenheim. "Husbands' Versus Wives' Fertility Goals and Use of Contraception: The Influence of Gender Context in Five Asian Countries." *Demography.* August 2000, 37:3, p. 299. A look at the way that gender conflict within families affects decisions to have children and to use contraception.

Waiz, Nashid Kamal. "Role of Education in the Use of Contraception." *Lancet.* December 2000, Vol. 356, p. S51. Education is considered central in women's decisions to use contraception.

Weber, Wim. "Dutch Baby Boom As Society Adjusts to Working Mothers." *The Lancet.* September 2, 2000, 356:9232, p. 837. Providing support for working women in the Netherlands means that such women are more likely to have children.

REPRODUCTIVE TECHNOLOGY

Newspapers and Magazines

Abbott, Charlotte. "Sex in the Future: The Reproductive Revolution and How It Will Change Us." *Publishers Weekly.* May 1, 2000, 247:18, p. 64. Book review.

———. "The Second Creation: Dolly and the Age of Biological Control." *Publishers Weekly.* April 17, 2000, 247:16, p. 59. Book review.

Alexander, Brian. "(You)^2." *Wired.* February 2001, 8:03, p. 220. An overview of the latest research on cloning.

Andrews, Lori. "No More Custom-Made Babies." *Self.* April 2000, 22:4, p. 128. Andrews has been one of the legal experts on reproductive technology; she now questions her previous support for certain types of fertility treatments as she sees where her efforts have led.

Annas, George J. "Conceiving One Child to Save Another; It Does Not Cross the Line, But Puts Us Very Near It." *Boston Globe.* October 15, 2000, p. C.1. The chair of the Health Law Department at the Boston University School of Public Health questions the decision of Jack and Lisa Nash, who used genetic techniques to create a child that could donate cells to their daughter, Molly, who suffered from Fanconi anemia.

Anstett, Patricia. "Blastocyst Transfer." *Chicago Tribune.* March 17, 2000, p. 7. Last year, a Michigan couple pioneers the use of blastocyst transfer, a new fertility technique designed to limit IVF babies to singletons and twins.

"Asch Is Gone—Now Move On." *Los Angeles Times.* July 29, 2000, p. 12. Drs. Ricardo Asch, Jose Balmaceda, and Sergio Stone were all involved in a fertility scandal at U.C. Irvine; the editorial analyzes the scandal and advises the university to move on.

Associated Press. "Bioethics Reports Criticizes Payments of More Than $10,000 for Ovarian Egg Donations." *St. Louis Post-Dispatch.* August 4, 2000, p. A.16. A bioethics report suggests that women donating eggs be paid a limited amount—and nowhere near the high figures that have been paid in recent months.

———. "No Visitation Rights for Couple in Embryo Mix-Up." (Albany) *Times Union.* October 27, 2000, p. A.10. An African-American couple is denied visitation rights to the white woman who gave birth to their biological child after a mix-up at a fertility clinic.

Auge, Karen. "Four of a Kind Parents Hit Jackpot With Quadruplets." *Denver Post.* October 17, 2000, p. A.01. A family's personal experience with having quadruplets, resulting from the IVF treatment of 40-year-old Sharon Molnar.

Bailey, Issac J. "Hundreds Say They Conceived After Touching Fertility Statues." *Houston Chronicle.* October 15, 2000, p. 25. Fertility statues in front of Ripley's "Believe It Or Not!" museum in Myrtle Beach, South Carolina, are attracting hundreds of women worldwide, who claim to have become pregnant after touching the statues.

Barbier, Sandra. "One-year-old Is the Engineered Cat's Meow; Center May Duplicate Breakthrough Baby." (New Orleans) *Times-Picayune.* November 24, 2001, p. 1. Jazz, an African wildcat at the Audubon Zoo in New Orleans, is the first animal born of an egg fertilized through IVF that was frozen, thawed, and transferred to a different species—in this case, a domestic cat. One year after birth, the "surrogate baby" wildcat is doing well.

Boseley, Sarah. "Stampede for IVF Puts Women at Risk, Says Expert." *Guardian.* June 29, 2000, p. 5. A Utrecht fertility specialist tells a conference that women are rushing to undergo IVF far too quickly, out of needless fears that they may be infertile.

Branigan, Tania. "Clinic Boss Defends Pregnant Woman, 56." *The Guardian.* January 23, 2001, p. 3. Ian Craft, of the London Gynaecology and Fertility Centre, defends his clinic's decision to treat a 56-year-old woman, who will become the oldest recorded mother of twins in Britain.

Bretting, Sandra. "Family, By the Numbers." *Houston Chronicle.* March 19, 2000, p. 4. The personal account of a woman with one child who is longing to have another, a desire that prompts her to seek the help of reproductive technology.

"Changing the Calculation." *St. Louis Post-Dispatch.* January 31, 2001, p. B.6. Italian fertility specialist Panayiotis M. Zavos announces the goal of cloning a human for an infertile couple within two years. Zavos had previously helped a 62-year-old women conceive a child.

Charen, Mona. "New Embryo Rules Portend a Harvesting of Human Life." *Detroit News.* August 27, 2000, p. 7. A look at the implications of new rules for stem-cell research.

Chase, Marilyn. "Doctors Begin Offering Creative Payment Plans for Fertility Treatment." *Wall Street Journal.* September 8, 2000, p. B.1. Some 50% of infertile couples never seek treatment, which doctors believe is primarily for financial reasons, so some fertility centers are now offering money-back plans and other incentives.

Coleman, Joshua. "Gender Vendors: Pro: The Pluses, More Choice, Fewer Unwanted Children." *San Francisco Chronicle.* October 1, 2000, p. 4.A.1. The "pro" side of a debate about using technology to determine a child's gender.

Reproductive Rights and Technology

"Couple Offers $100,000 in Ad Seeking Woman to Donate Eggs." *Los Angeles Times.* February 9, 2000, p. A.20. An ad offering $100,000 for the eggs of a "bright, young, white athlete" may be the highest offer yet made for human eggs.

Curwen, Thomas. "Book Review: Where Miracle of Life Collides With Forces of Nature; BABY E.R. The Heroic Doctors and Nurses Who Perform Medicine's Tiniest Miracles; by Edward Humes." *Los Angeles Times.* January 18, 2001, p. E.3. A review of a book about the heroic measures available to save premature babies.

Davies, Saffron. "Science: The Chemical Generation: Have Man-Made Chemicals Affected Our Fertility?" *The Guardian.* November 2, 2000, p. 2. A look at how fertility has been affected by the more than 80,000 synthetic chemicals in everyday use.

Davis, Bob. "Put to the Test: GOP Avoids Abortion for Now, but Science is Stirring the Debate—Research that Kills Embryos But May Fight Diseases Prompts Reassessments—A Senator and His Conscience." *Wall Street Journal.* August 1, 2000, p. A.1. Antiabortion legislators may not vote against stem-cell research.

Davis, Katherine. "Is Natural Birth Control Better?" *Self.* December 2000, 22:12, p. 82. A look at whether natural family planning is effective.

Dunn, Jancee. "Melissa's Secret." *Rolling Stone.* February 3, 2000, Issue 833, p. 40. Rock star Melissa Etheridge and her partner, filmmaker Julie Cypher, reveal that the father of their baby is David Crosby, founding member of the Byrds and Crosby, Stills and Nash.

Dyer, Clare. "Fertility Clinic Sued for Unwanted Third Baby: Couple May Get Pounds 100,000 After 'Shock' of Having Triplets." *The Guardian.* November 15, 2000, p. 5. A couple sues a fertility clinic after unexpectedly having triplets.

Ellement, John. "SJC Explains Fertility Treatment Decision." *Boston Globe.* April 1, 2000, p. B.3. Massachusetts' highest court ruled that courts will not support "forced procreation," forcing people to become parents against their will; the Supreme Judicial Court defends its decision of earlier this year to refuse a woman's request to be implanted with four embryos from her failed marriage.

———. "SJC Rules in Embryo Case; Man Wins Bid to Bar Their Use by Ex-wife." *Boston Globe.* February 10, 2000, p. B.1. The Massachusetts Supreme Judicial Court rules that a woman cannot implant embryos created during her failed marriage if her ex-husband no longer wants to become a parent.

Emmons, Jim. "Treating Male Infertility, Syracuse Urologist Says Many Couples Fail to See the Need for the Man to Be Tested." (Syracuse) *Post-Standard.* July 31, 2000, p. C.1. A doctor warns that men, as well as women, should be tested when a couple is infertile.

Annotated Bibliography

Errico-Cox, Lisa A. "Six Steps to Increased Fertility: An Integrated Mind/Body and Medical Program to Promote Conception." *Library Journal.* September 1, 2000, 125:14, p. 239. Book review.

"Ethical Rules for Stem Cell Research." *Boston Globe.* August 27, 2000, p. F.6. An editorial advocating stem-cell research.

"Fecundity of Males Is Found to Decline After the Age of 24." *Wall Street Journal.* August 29, 2000, p. B.7.A. A new study reveals that women are not the only ones whose fertility declines with age.

"Fertility Cut by Passive Smoking." *The Guardian.* September 30, 2000, p. 14. A longitudinal study finds that nonsmoking women exposed to smoke increases by 14 percent the odds of taking more than twelve months to conceive.

Feuer, Alan. "Two More Men Are Charged in a Mob Killing in 1988." *New York Times.* November 29, 2000, p. B.3. While Mafia figure George Zappola ("Georgie Neck") was in prison, he arranged to have his sperm smuggled out, so that when he was released from prison, he would find a grown child waiting for him; the woman who was to carry Zappola's child changed her mind and cooperated with federal agents instead.

Fox, Michael J. "A Crucial Election for Medical Research." *New York Times.* November 1, 2000, p. A.35. The actor Michael J. Fox, who has Parkinson's disease, argues that stem-cell research should proceed, as it may help cure many devastating illnesses. Fox claims that although stem-cell research involves cells extracted from embryos, it differs from fetal tissue research and should not alarm right-to-life advocates.

Freely, Maureen. "Parents2: Never Say Never: New Evidence Indicates That Older Women May Be Jeopardising the Health of Their Children by Leaving Motherhood Late. Nonsense, Says Maureen Freely." *Guardian.* October 4, 2000, p. 8. The author looks skeptically at studies that criticize older mothers for putting their children's health in jeopardy.

Friedman, Lyssa. "Out of the Cabbage Patch, Into the Lab." *San Francisco Chronicle.* October 1, 2000, p. 4.A.1. A look at technologies used to determine the gender of a child.

Gauen, Pat. "A Close Calls Turns Tears of Sadness to Tears of Joy." *St. Louis Post-Dispatch.* August 21, 2000, p. 2. A personal account of a doctor who managed to save a pregnancy by averting the D&C of a baby mistakenly believed to have miscarried.

Goodman, Ellen. "A Blessed Event—At What Price?" *Boston Globe.* October 8, 2000, p. D.7. The columnist looks critically at the birth of Adam Nash, the first child conceived with the help of genetic tests to be a cell donor for another person—in this case, his six-year-old sister, Molly. Goodman is concerned about the possibility of "designer babies."

————. "When Fertility Is a Pre-Existing Condition." (Albany) *Times Union.* July 28, 2000, p. A.15. A look at a class-action suit trying to obtain insurance coverage for contraceptives.

Gosden, Roger. "New Options for Mothers." *The Futurist.* March/April 2000, 34:2, p. 26. A discussion of the best methods of procreation for post-menopausal women.

Grady, Denise. "Son Conceived to Provide Blood Cells for Daughter." *New York Times.* October 4, 2000, p. A.24. Adam Nash, born on August 29, is the first child specifically conceived with the help of genetic tests to produce a baby with the traits needed for a sibling's cell transplant.

Greenberg, Noah. "How Old Is Too Old to Have a Baby." *Discover.* April 2000, 21:4, p. 60. A look at technology that may make it possible for older men and post-menopausal women to have children.

Grigoriades, Vanessa. "Being a Sperm Donor Is Hard Work." *Rolling Stone.* October 26, 2000, Issue 852, p. 77. Interviews with several college-age sperm donors enliven an account of the donation process.

Hartill, Lane. "What's New for Sale on International Market—Human Sperm." *Christian Science Monitor.* January 13, 2000, p. 14. International trade in human sperm is growing quickly but quietly.

Illescas, Carlos. "For Molly, 6, So Far, So Good; Umbilical Blood From Baby Brother Seems to Be Working, Doctors Tell Her Parents." *Denver Post.* October 19, 2000, p. B.01. Molly Nash, suffering from Fanconi anemia, is doing well after receiving a treatment from her brother Adam's umbilical blood. Adam was conceived with the help of genetic tests that determined his suitability as a donor for Molly.

Jackson, Irvin L. "Livingston Kidnap Suspect Is Extradited; Local Mom Acused of Stealing Her Son Is Pregnant Again." *Detroit News.* October 25, 2000, p. 1. Sarah Bohn and Michael Mobley are embroiled in a legal battle over embryos that the two of them created and stored at an Ann Arbor fertility clinic; Mobley wants the embryos destroyed while Bohn wants to bear the children.

"Jury Convicts Fertility Doctor of Defrauding Insurance Firms." *Houston Chronicle.* January 20, 2001, p. 13. Dr. Niels Lauersen is convicted of defrauding insurance companies, whom he billed for surgeries that never took place. Instead, Lauersen provided women with fertility treatments while pocketing $2.5 million illegally between 1987 and 1997.

Kamata, Suzanne. "Multiple Choice." *Utne Reader.* September/October 2000, Issue 101, p. 42. The author describes the abortion that she had at age 20, which damaged her reproductive system. She later undergoes IVF and then must decide whether to selectively reduce the fetuses she is carrying so as to increase her chances of a successful birth.

Kelly, Alice Lesch. "Does Stress Hurt Fertility?" *Joe Weider's Shape.* 22:1, p. 18. A mind-body infertility program offered by Beth Israel Deaconess Medical Center in Boston claims that decreasing stress can increase fertility.

Konigsberg, Eric. "The Ob-Gyn Who Loves Women." *New York.* June 19, 2000, 33:24, p. 24. Dr. Niels Lauersen, awaiting a retrial for insurance fraud, is defended by dozens of patients during state and federal investigations. Lauersen had billed insurance companies for surgeries that never took place while providing his patients with fertility treatments instead.

Kotulak, Ronald, and Jon Van. "Discoveries." *Chicago Tribune.* January 30, 2000, p. 13.3. From 1994 to 1998, the success rate for IVF increased from 14.9 percent to 22.5 percent, according to a report by Dr. Daniel W. Cramer reported in the journal *Obstetrics & Gynecology.*

Kreck, Carol. "Preemie Births Can Be Avoided; Moms Must Quit Smoking, Gain Weight." *Denver Post.* September 29, 2000. p. A.01. If all pregnant women gained sufficient weight and avoided smoking, low-birth-weight rates in Colorado could be reduced by 25%, according to a new study.

Kuzemchak, Sally. "What's the Best Birth Control for You?" *American Baby.* September 2000, 62:9, p. 64. A look at the available methods of birth control for a new mother.

Landler, Mark. "Clinic Caters to Couples Seeking 'Precious Gem.'" *New York Times.* July 1, 2000, p. A.4. Anthony S. Y. Wong's fertility clinic in Hong Kong offers a chance for parents to choose the sex of their prospective children.

Laurence, Leslie. "The Hidden Health Threat That Puts Every Woman At Risk." *Redbook.* July 2000, 195:1, p. 112. A report on the 132 nonsectarian hospitals that merged with Catholic hospitals from 1995–2000 and the trend's implications for reproductive rights.

Leland, John. "O.K., You're Gay. So? Where's My Grandchild?" *New York Times.* December 21, 2000, p. F1. A look at how the new acceptance of gay and lesbian couples is leading to pressure from prospective grandparents.

Leonard, Mary. "Abortion Foes See Politics in Stem-Cell Study Policy." *Boston Globe.* August 24, 2000, p. A.1. Abortion opponents are critical of new federal guidelines of stem-cell research.

Lewin, Tamar. "Report Links Fertility Aids to Small Size in Newborns." *New York Times.* July 15, 2000, p. A.7. A look at the dangerous increase in low-birth-weight babies and the trend's relationship to ART.

Macleod, Alexander. "Twins Test Limits of British Law; A Gay British Couple's Plan to Raise their US-Born Twins Challenged." *Christian Science Monitor.* January 13, 2000, p. 6. Two male partners—one of whom is the biological father of twins—are engaged in a legal dispute with British authorities over their status as parents.

Magill, Gerard. "Stem Cell Controversy Shows the Need to Bridge Science and Ethics." *St. Louis Post-Dispatch.* September 3, 2000, p. B.3. The director of the Center for Health Care Ethics at St. Louis University discusses the stem-cell research controversy.

Malcolm, Teresa. "Women Battle Bishops Over Reproductive Technology." *National Catholic Reporter.* November 10, 2000, 37:4, p. 8. An Australian feminist group challenges their country's Catholic bishops over the rights of lesbian and single mothers to reproductive technology.

Malmstrom, Patricia Maxwell. "Gender Vendors, Con: The Downside: Babies Will Become Commodities." *San Francisco Chronicle.* October 1, 2000, p. 4.Z.1. The "con" side in a debate over using technology to select the sex of unborn children.

Marosi, Richard. "Fertility Doctor's Case May See Delays; Extraditing Dr. Jose P. Balmaceda, Wanted in '94 UC Irvine Scandal, Could Take a Year in Argentina." *Los Angeles Times.* January 23, 2001. Jose P. Balmaceda is accused of mail fraud and tax evasion because of a supposed scheme to defraud insurance companies for fertility treatments while he allegedly harvested eggs from women and either implanted them in other women or used them for research.

Marquis, Julie. "Court Limits Anonymity of Sperm Donors." *Los Angeles Times.* May 20, 2000, p. 1. A California appellate court rules that an anonymous sperm donor does not have an unlimited right to privacy but can be forced to testify in legal actions alleging that his sperm resulted in genetic harm to a child.

Marx, Patricia. "Perfect Specimen." *Vogue.* August 2000, 190:8, p. 168. An account of a visit to Fairfax Cryobank, one of the world's largest human sperm banks; the author explores the personal profiles of sperm donors.

McDonald, Maureen. "Happy Parents Make Adoption Lawyer's Day; She Knows Firsthand About the Joy, Pain of Building a Family." *Detroit News.* December 22, 2000, p. 2. Lawyer Monica Farris Linkner specializes in issues involving adoption and reproductive technology.

Meikle, James. "Three Embryos 'Too Many' for IVF Treatment: Multiple Births Caused by Couples Stacking Odds: The Background: Fertility." *Guardian.* November 17, 2000, p. A 1. An article exploring the connection between fertility treatments and multiple births.

"Multiple Births Not Necessarily a Consequence of Conception Drugs." *USA Today.* February 2000, 128:2657, p. 15. A report by Serono Laboratories says that fertility drugs result in multiple births of three or more babies in fewer than 6% of all cases.

Nagourney, Eric. "New Findings on Fallopian Implants." *New York Times.* November 14, 2000, p. F.8. Contrary to other reports, two methods of IVF have about the same success rate, according to a study by Dr. Steven Palter of the Yale School of Medicine.

Nelson, Kathleen, "SLU Coach Nolen Doesn't Need to Recruit Help for Her New Twins." *St. Louis Post-Dispatch.* September 29, 2000, p. B.1. A look at St. Louis University coach Marilyn Nolen, who gave birth to twins at the age of 55.

"Of Mice, Jellyfish & Us." *Commonweal.* January 28, 2000, 127:2, p. 5. An article raising questions about the ethics of genetic manipulation.

Pappert, Ann. "What Price Pregnancy." *Ms.* June/July 2000, 10:4, p. 42. Scientist are finding some proof that fertility drugs may cause ovarian cancer.

Parker, Kathleen. "Baby Case Ends with Multiracial Scrambled Eggs." *Chicago Tribune.* June 21, 2000, p. 17. The author speculates about a case in which woman is implanted with someone else's egg.

Pedersen, Kelly. "Fourteen Candles: Surviving Seven Chukwu Octuplets Turn 2 Years Old." *Houston Chronicle.* December 21, 2000, p. 33. A look at life in the Chukwu family of Houston, where seven surviving octuplets have turned two years old. Chukwu was taking fertility drugs when she conceived first triplets, who died stillborn or soon after birth, and then octuplets, seven of whom survived. She is the only known woman to give birth to eight living babies.

Pertman, Adam. "Sidebar: A Life Story With a New Twist." *Boston Globe.* August 8, 2000, p. E.1. The profile of a couple who adopted an embryo.

Pinkerton, James P. "Commentary: The Story Now Delivers a Stark Reality." *Los Angeles Times.* January 2, 2001, p. B7. An editorial warning that upper-income women are having fewer children, as lower-income women are having more; the author invokes Darwin's theories to explain why this is dangerous.

Poblete, Pati. "We Should Reset Priorities, Not Nature's Clock." *San Francisco Chronicle.* September 10, 2000, p. 5.Z.1. Dr. Roger Gosden wants to delay menopause, but the author would rather see society making it easier for women to have children at earlier ages.

Press Association. "Home Appliances 'Impair Fertility.'" *Guardian.* October 31, 2000, p. 10. An Italian study in the journal *Human Reproduction* suggests that exposure to radiation from electrical appliances and power lines may make women infertile.

Radford, Tim. "Scientists Predict Stem Cell Trials by 2004." *Guardian.* January 24, 2001, p. 10. Stem cells taken from human embryos may soon be used to treat Parkinson's disease.

Recer, Paul. "Funding for Research of Embryo Cells OK'd." *Denver Post.* August 24, 2000, p. A.15. A report on research showing that stem cells may be able to restore nerve tissue and some functioning in mice following stroke or spinal cord injury.

"Report Suggests Limits on Pay for Egg Donors." *New York Times.* August 5, 2000, p. A.9. The ethics committee of the American Society for Reproductive Medicine recommends a limit on how much egg donors should be paid.

Rigali, Norbert J. "Words and Contraception." *America*. September 23, 2000, 183:8, p. 8. The Roman Catholic Church needs to clarify what kinds of human control of fertility are morally responsible.

Ritter, Malcolm. "Science Uncovering the Why of the 'Y'; Gene Work May Give Male Fertility Insight." *Houston Chronicle*. October 31, 2000, p. 11. A look at some of the latest research into male fertility issues.

Rosenwaks, Zev. "We Still Can't Stop the Biological Clock." *New York Times*. June 24, 2000, p. A.15. The director of the Center for Reproductive Medicine and Infertility at New York-Presbyterian Hospital-Weill Cornell Campus warns of the dangers of older women believing that they can conceive and give birth at any age.

Ross, Emma. "Men Have a Biological Clock, Too; Study: Males Past Age 24 Take Longer to Make Babies." *Denver Post*. August 1, 2000, p. A.1. A new study shows that men's age is involved in fertility.

Rotella, Mark. "The Elusive Embryo: How Men and Women Approach New Reproductive Technologies." *Publishers Weekly*. November 20, 2000, 247:47, p. 60. Book review.

Rubin, Alissa J., and Aaron Zitner. "Infertility Cases Spur an Illicit Drug Market: Health: Women Buy Leftover Fertility Medication From Other Patients, Often Online, But Law Enforcement Is Lax." *Los Angeles Times*. September 10, 2000, p. 1. Women who cannot afford to pay for infertility drugs and do not have insurance coverage have begun seeking their medications on the Internet.

Rubin, Rita. "Intelligence and Good Health Top the Savvy Parent Shopper's List." *USA Today*. November 2, 2000, p. D.1. A look at the Fairfax Cryobank, a popular sperm bank.

———. "Tied Tubes Don't Upset Menstrual Cycle." *USA Today*. December 7, 2000, p. 9D. More than 10 million U.S. women and more than 100 million women worldwide have had their tubes tied according to a study conducted by Herbert Peterson and others; his study refutes the long-held idea that tubal ligation causes menstrual problems.

———. "Who's My Father? Progeny Seeks Some Conception of Sperm Donors." *USA Today*. November 2, 2000, p. 1. D. For many years, sperm donors' identities were kept secret, but now sperm banks offer information about donors and in some cases, make it possible for donors and offspring to find each other.

Sapp, Gregg. "The Clone Age: Adventures in the New World of Reproductive Technology." *Library Journal*. March 1, 2000, 125:4, p. 56. Book review.

Schulman, Audrey. "Inconceivable." *Ms.* June/July 2000, 10:4, p. 50. A skeptical and personal look at fertility treatments, in which the author describes how both she and her sister were treated differently by fertility doctors than their husbands were: Medical technology was mobilized to treat women with extensive, invasive procedures, as the men were virtually ignored.

Sottile, Beverly. "Cover Infertility Treatment Instead of Contraceptives." *Buffalo News.* September 23, 2000, p. B.6. In response to Ellen Goodman's column calling for insurance coverage of contraceptives, the author claims that infertility treatments are more deserving of coverage.

Spiker, Ted. "Oh, Baby, Baby." *Men's Health.* January/February 2001, 16:1, p. 40. A look at a recent study finding that men having more satisfying sex were more likely to have a higher sperm count—and so were more likely to fertilize their partners.

Stanley, Alessandra. "Couple Leave Italy After Rebuff Over Surrogate Motherhood." *New York Times.* May 11, 2000, p. A.13. An anonymous Italian couple battled Italy's medical establishment and legal system, winning a judge's approval for surrogate motherhood when the Italian Medical Association blocked their doctor from performing the procedure. When the case continued to be appealed, the couple decided to leave Italy.

Steinhauer, Jennifer, and Sherri Day. "Doctor Convicted of Insurance Fraud in Fertility Procedures." *New York Times.* January 10, 2001, p. B.1. Dr. Niels Lauersen is convicted of insurance fraud; the doctor got insurance companies to pay for expensive—and noncovered—fertility procedures by billing them for nonexistent surgeries instead.

Steinhauer, Jennifer. "Mistrial for Fertility Doctor Accused of Insurance Fraud." *New York Times.* March 7, 2000, p. B.7. The seven-week trial of Dr. Niels H. Lauersen ends in mistrial. Lauersen was indicted for billing insurers for surgery to mask his true activities: providing fertility treatment to female patients. In the process, law enforcement officials said, he brought in approximately $4 million.

Stolberg, Sheryl Gay. "Stem Cell Research Advocates in Limbo." *New York Times.* January 20, 2001, p. A.17. Stem-cell research holds promise for the treatment of human diseases, but pro-life activists consider the research immoral, as stem cells come from human embryos.

Stovsky, Renee. "A Webster Grove Couple Go Through Their Own Baby Boom." *St. Louis Post-Dispatch.* May 15, 2000, p. E.1. A look at Barbara and Dan Wright, a Missouri couple who had triplets after Barbara received fertility treatments.

Stream, Carol. "Thus Spoke Superman." *Christianity Today.* June 12, 2000, 44:7, p. 33. Actor Christopher Reeve advocates stem-cell research, but the author argues that a Christian perspective would consider this a callous disregard for human life.

Struck, Doug. "Japanese Preserve Bloodlines; Grandfather's Sperm Used for Conception." *Houston Chronicle.* November 18, 2000, p. 34. Japan has embraced modern fertility techniques slowly, but some procedures are becoming more common, while others are shunned.

Stryker, Jeff. "Take It to the Bank." *New York Times Magazine.* June 25, 2000, p. 20. The history of sperm banking from the 1950s to the present, and a look at the growing demand for artificial insemination in the United States.

Stukin, Stacie. "The Scramble for Eggs." *Glamour.* February 2000, 98:2, p. 218. Ron's Angels is a web site that auctions the eggs of beautiful women to the highest bidders; this article takes a closer look at the controversy.

Tarkan, Laurie. "Last-Minute Motherhood." *McCall's.* March 2000, 127:6, p. 36. A look at three women who became pregnant for the first time after the age of 40.

Toolis, Kevin. "Comment & Analysis: Hate That Dare Not Speak Its Name: Behind Yesterday's Fresh Courtroom Clashes in the Case of the Conjoined Twins Lies Our Secret Prejudice." *Guardian.* September 15, 2000, p. 20. A critique of what the author sees as the British media's biased treatment of conjoined twins in a controversy over separating two such twins.

Torassa, Ulysses. "Marijuana May Hurt Couples' Conception Odds/Studies Find Fertilization Inhibited by Compound That Resembles Cannabis." *San Francisco Chronicle.* December 13, 2000, p. A.9. New research raises the possibility that using marijuana may impair a couple's chances of becoming pregnant.

Trafford, Abigail. "Second Opinion: Miracle Babies Draw Us Into an Ethical Swamp." *Washington Post.* November 14, 2000, p. Z.8. An editorial raising questions about the ethics of the birth of Adam Nash, who was conceived with the help of genetic tests that showed he could donate cells to his sister, Molly, suffering from Fanconi anemia.

Truitt, Eliza. "Egg Donation: A Risky Business." *Rolling Stone.* October 26, 2000, Issue 852, p. 80. A look at the risks of egg donation, including the possibilty of ovarian cancer from the fertility drugs used in the process.

Vajjhala, Surekha. "When Stork Fever Hits; A Sobering Look at the Dangers of Fertility Drugs." *U.S. News & World Report.* July 17, 2000, p. 1. A study in the *New England Journal of Medicine* finds that the use of injectable hormones stimulating the release of eggs creates an "unacceptable risk" of pregnancy with three or more fetuses.

VandeWater, Judith. "Fertility Doctors Use Advertising and Refund Offers to Woo Couples; Pricing Packages, Money-Back Guarantees and Unconventional Methods Have Caused Some Physicians to Become Concerned for Patients' Health." *St. Louis Post-Dispatch.* February 5, 2001, p. 10. A look at the growing commercialization of fertility clinics.

————. "Most Insurers Won't Cover the Cost of Fertility Treatment; Going Through One Round of Procedures Can Cost as Much as $15,000." *St. Louis Post-Dispatch*, February 5, 2001, p. 10.

————. "There Are Low-Tech Ways to Improve Fertility, Too." *St. Louis Post-Dispatch.* February 5, 2001, p. 12. An account of registered nurse Beck Kubala, founder of P.A.R.I.N.T.S., a Missouri fertility clinic that focuses on low-tech treatments.

Vergano, Dan. "In-vitro Selection Could Save a Sibling." *USA Today.* October 5, 2000, p. 11.D. Coverage of Lisa and Jack Nash's decision to conceive a child that might donate umbilical-cord blood to their fatally ill daughter.

Wade, Nicholas. "U.S. to Pay for Embryo Stem Cell Research; New Rules Set Limits for Use of Tissue Taken from Fertility Clinics." *Chicago Tribune.* August 24, 2000, p. 20. Recent experiments have shown that stem-cell research has exciting possibilities; a look at new federal rules for the research.

Wainwright, Martin. "I Never Agreed to Treatment, Says Triplets Case Wife." *Guardian.* November 16, 2000, p. 8. Coverage of a suit against a fertility clinic brought by a British couple who gave birth to triplets.

Warshall, Peter. "High-Tech Conception: A Comprehensive Handbook for Consumers." *Whole Earth.* Summer 2000, Issue 101, p. 13. Book review.

Wasserstein, Wendy. "Annals of Motherhood: Complications." *New Yorker.* February 21–February 28, 2000, 76:1, p. 87. A detailed personal account of the difficulties that the author—an award-winning playwright and single mother—faced during her pregnancy.

Weiss, Kenneth R. "California and the West; UC Regents Fire Professor Involved in Fertility Case; Education: UC Irvine Clinic Physician, Who Fled U.S. to Avoid Charges, Was Accused of Stealing Human Eggs and Embryos." *Los Angeles Times.* July 21, 2000, p. 3. A response to the scandal involving Dr. Ricardo Asch, who was accused of stealing human eggs and embryos that were implanted in women without their knowledge or used for research without the donor's consent.

Weiss, Rick. "British Panel Urges Allowing Human Embryo Cloning; Proposal Would Put Country in Forefront of Stem Cell Research—and at the Center of Controversy." *Washington Post.* August 17, 2000, p. A.26. A British science and ethics commission recommended that British researchers should be allowed to clone human embryos for research purposes as long as the embryos are destroyed within two weeks.

————. "Embryo Test May Aid Fertility Treatment." *Denver Post.* October 23, 2000, p. A.1. Researchers have developed a new test that can examine each chromosome of a three-day-old human test-tube embryo—a test that might improve success rates at fertility clinics.

———. "Gene-tinkering Yields Modified Monkey." (Albany) *Times Union.* January 12, 2001, p. A1. Fertility clinics already allow parents to "design" their babies to some extent; a gene-altered monkey born in Oregon in October 2000 opens the possibility of further genetic manipulation of human children.

———. "Human Cloning's 'Numbers Game': Technology Puts Breakthrough Within the Reach of Sheer Persistence." *Washington Post.* October 10, 2000, p. A.1. A look at Clonaid, a human cloning company run by a Canadian religious sect called the Raelians.

———. "Limited Pay for Egg Donors Advised: Report Proposes a Variety of Other Ethical Standards for Infertility Treatment." *Washington Post.* August 4, 2000, p. A.5. A medical ethics committee recomends that women who donate their eggs for fertility treatments should be paid—but only rarely more than $5,000 and never as much as $10,000.

———. "U.S. Fertility Expert Announces Effort to Clone a Human; Consortium Led by Renegade Doctor Says It Will Help Infertile Couples." *Washington Post.* January 27, 2001, p. A3. Panos Zavos, founder of a Lexington fertility clinic, plans to collaborate with Italian fertility doctor Severino Antinori to produce a cloned baby within 12 to 24 months.

Weller, Sheila. "The Online Fertility Drug Trade." *Self.* July 2000, 22:7, p. 72. The high price of fertility drugs has led to a brisk online trade among sometimes desperate couples seeking help in having children.

Whitney, Daisy. "The Baby Business; Donor Eggs Give Women Chance to Bear Children." *Denver Post.* April 25, 2000, p. E.1. Egg donation is becoming a big business, with fees for eggs rising as high as $15,000 in some cases.

———. "In Vitro Process Works for Some." *Denver Post.* April 25, 2000, p. E1. A personal account of a woman's experience with IVF.

Zachary, G. Pascal. "A Most Unlikely Industry Finds It Can't Resist Globalization's Call—Exporting Human Sperm Is a Fast-Growth Business, Banks in Denmark, U.S. Find." *Wall Street Journal.* January 6, 2000, p. B1. Sperm banks discover that international demand for certain types of sperm—particularly from blue-eyed donors—is growing rapidly.

Zitner, Aaron. "Column One: Cold War in Fertility Technology; With More People Freezing Embryos for Future Use, Science Has Outpaced the Legal System. New Uses Are Emerging, and Debate Is Growing About How Human the Cell Clusters Are." *Los Angeles Times.* October 16, 2000, p. A.1. New legal and ethical questions have arisen about how to handle the estimated 100,000 human embryos currently being stored at fertility clinics.

Annotated Bibliography

Specialized Journals

Ashraf, Haroun. "UK Allows Frozen Eggs for Fertility Treatment." *Lancet.* January 29, 2000, 355:9201, p. 387. The UK Human Fertilisation and Embryology Authority annonces that frozen eggs may now be thawed and used by a London fertility clinic; previously, eggs could be frozen and stored, but not thawed and used.

Ayoub, Nina. "Nota Bene: Reproducing Jews; A Cultural Account of Assisted Conception in Israel." *Chronicle of Higher Education.* November 17, 2000, 47:12, p. A26. A review of the book, *Reproducing Jews: A Cultural Account of Assisted Conception in Israel,* by Martha Kahn, which allows the author to explore the responses of Orthodox rabbies to new reproductive technologies.

Baker, Debra. "Model Act on Hold." *ABA Journal.* June 2000, Vol. 86, p. 105. The American Bar Association Section of Family Law postponed endorsing a model act to regulate ART.

Beyzarov, Elena Portyansky. "New GnRH Antagonist May Simplify Fertility Regimens." *Drug Topics.* October 2, 2000, 144:19, p. 28. A new hormone released onto the market may enable new and simpler forms of ovulation induction.

Blacksher, Erika. "A Request for ICSI/Commentary. *The Hastings Center Report.* March/April 2000, 30:2, p. 23. An account of a case involving an HIV-positive man and an HIV-negative woman seeking to get pregnant via ICSI, a treatment that may be safer procedure when HIV is involved.

———. "On Ova Commerce." *The Hastings Center Report,* September/October 2000, 30:5, p. 29. The author considers the question of selling her eggs and concludes that some things belong outside the realm of commerce.

Briggs, Laura. "'There Is Not Unauthorized Breeding in Jurassic Park;' Gender and the Uses of Genetics." *NWSA Journal.* Fall 2000, 12:3, p. 92. A close reading of the book and the movie *Jurassic Park* and the movie *Gattaca* show that popular culture draws upon profound antifeminism.

Burks, Deborah H. "IRS-2 Pathways Integrate Female Reproduction and Energy Homeostasis." *Nature.* September 21, 2000. 407:6802, p. 377. Severe restrictions on diet can interfere with mammals' fertility, and obesity may be associated with various infertile conditions, including polycystic ovary syndrome.

"Contribution of Assisted Reproduction Technology and Ovulation-Inducing Drugs to Triplet and Higher-Order Multiple Births—United States 1980–1987." *JAMA.* July 19, 2000, 284:3, p. 299. U.S. pregnancies resulting from ART are more likely to result in multiple births than unassisted reproduction; and triplets or higher-order births are at greater risk than the birth of singletons.

"Contribution of Assisted Reproduction Technology and Ovulation-Inducing Drugs to Triplet and Higher-Order Multiple Births—United States 1980–1987." *MMWR*, June 23, 2000, 49:24, p. 535. The rate of triplets and high-order multiple births has more than quadrupled, largely due to ART and ovulation-inducing drugs.

Cooper, W.H. "The Psychological Predictors of Pain During IVF Egg Retrieval." *Journal of Reproductive and Infant Psychology*. May 2000, 18:2, p. 97. A study of 34 women undergoing the egg retrieval commonly used in IVF treatment, finding that women experienced relatively high levels of pain.

Daniels, K.R. "To Give or Sell Human Gametes—The Interplay Between Pragmatics, Policy and Ethics." *Journal of Medical Ethics*. June 2000, 26:3, p. 206. A discussion of the ethics of paying for sperm and eggs to be used in various fertility treatments.

Day, Michael. "Mice to the Rescue." *New Scientist*. July 1, 2000, 167:2245, p. 7.

Docimo, Steven G. "The Undescended Testicle: Diagnosis and Management." *American Family Physician*. November 1, 2000, 62:9, p. 2037. The article argues that early diagnosis and management of an undescended testicle is crucial to improve fertility and to help detect malignancies.

Dunson, David B. "A Bayesian Model of Fecundability and Sterility." *Journal of the American Statistical Association*. December 2000, 95:452, p. 1054. A discussion of the role that environmental toxins play in decreased fertility.

"Even Second-hand Smoke Impairs Fertility." *Better Nutrition*. December 2000, 62:12, p. 22. According to a study of more than 14,000 pregnancies published in the medical journal *Fertility and Sterility*, women exposed to secondhand smoke were 15% less likely to conceive within 12 months as those in smoke-free surroundings.

Feng, Yi. "The Politics of Fertility and Economic Development." *International Studies Quarterly*. December 2000, 44:4, p. 667. An exploration of how political factors affect fertility decisions.

"First NDIF Baby Born to Infertile Woman in Minnesota." *PR Newswire*. October 19, 2000, p. 1. Coverage of a company that offers a nonsurgical solution to tubal infertility.

Fishman, Rachelle H.B. "Israel Faces Changes in IVF Regulation." *Lancet*. June 3, 2000, 355:9219, p. 1979. Israel seems to be liberalizing its policy on fertility treatments and egg donation.

Foubister, Vida. "Reproductive Technologies Outpacing Ethical Considerations." *American Medical News*. January 17, 2000, 43:2, p. 7. The author argues that ethics are being disregarded as individuals are offered new reproductive technologies and calls for more regulation of the fertility industry.

George, Susan A. "Not Exactly 'Of Woman Born': Procreation and Creation in Recent Science Fiction Films." *Journal of Popular Film & Television.* Winter 2001, 28:4, p. 176. A look at *Gattaca, Species,* and *Mimic,* three films with images of procreation; the author finds the genetic engineering holds both promise and fear for modern viewers.

Gerstein, L. "Maternal Factors and Multiple Births Are Main Cause of Poor Birth Outcomes After In Vitro Fertilization." *Family Planning Perspectives.* May/June 2000, 32:3, p. 149. Statistics showing the association of IVF with multiple births, based on a Swedish study that found that the rate of multiple pregnancies among IVF women was 27%, as opposed to only 1% of the general population.

Goslinga-Roy, Gillian M. "Body Boundaries, Fiction of the Female Self: An Ethnographic Perspective on Power, Feminism, and the Reproductive Technologies." *Feminist Studies.* Spring 2000, 26:1, p. 113. The author, an anthropologist, followed a couple that sponsored a surrogate mother, interviewing all three parties to the surrogate pregnancy. She concludes that many ideas about women's bodies and motherhood are viewed as "natural," but are in reality socially constructed and may be changed more easily than we suspect.

Gottlieb, Scott. "In Vitro Fertilisation Is Preferable to Fertility Drugs." *British Medical Journal.* July 15, 2000, 321:7254, p. 134. A study showing that inducing ovulation to treat infertility is likely to result in multiple births; therefore, the authors argue, IVF is preferable to using fertility drugs.

Gray, Ronald H. "Subfertility and Risk of Spontaneous Abortion." *American Journal of Public Health.* September 2000, 90:9, p. 1452. Subfertile women seem to experience an increased number of spontaneous abortions.

Hogan, Dennis P. "Sexual and Fertility Behaviors of American Females Aged 15–19 Years: 1985, 1990, and 1995." *American Journal of Public Health.* September 2000, 90:9, p. 1421. A study of changes in sexual and reproductive behavior from 1985 to 1995 among American 15- to 19-year-old girls. The trend toward teenaged motherhood has ended as young women are less sexually active and birth has control has become better; the most significant change, however, is improved family situations.

Hollander, D. "Fertility Drugs Do Not Raise Breast, Ovarian or Uterine Cancer Risk." *Family Planning Perspectives.* March/April 2000, 32:2, p. 100. A look at research suggesting that women who take fertility drugs in conjunction with IVF are not at increased risk of breast, ovarian, or uterine cancer; however, women who seek treatment but do not take fertility drugs are more than twice as much at risk for uterine cancer.

Kideckel, David A. "The Politics of Duplicity: Controlling Reproduction in Ceaucescu's Romania." *American Anthropologist.* March 2000, 102:1, p. 199. Book review.

Langdridge, D. "Reasons for Wanting a Child: A Network Analytic Study." *Journal of Reproductive and Infant Psychology.*" November 2000, 18:4, p. 321. A study exploring why couples want to be parents, comparing pregnant couples, couples seeking IVF, and couples seeking donor insemination.

Larkin, Marilynn. "Curb Costs of Egg Donation, Urge US Specialists." *Lancet.* August 23, 2000, 356:9299, p. 569. The American Society for Reproductive Medicine's ethics committee has advocated putting a limit on the fees that egg donors should be paid.

Ludwig, Michael. "In-vitro Fertilisation: A Future With No Limits?" *Lancet.* December 2000, 356, p. S52. A look at the possibilities and limits of IVF.

Martin, Steven P. "Diverging Fertility Among U.S. Women Who Delay Childbearing Past Age 30." *Demography.* November 2000, 37:4, p. 523. A look at the way that education affects women's decisions to have children.

Mayor, Susan. "Researchers Able to Check Chromosome Numbers in Embryos." *British Medical Journal.* October 28, 2000, 321:7268, p. 1040. A new technique for improving the rates of successful pregnancies with ART is discussed and analyzed.

McCoy, Norma L. "Women and New Reproductive Technologies: Medical, Psychosocial, Legal, and Ethical Dilemmas." *Archives of Sexual Behavior.* June 2000, 29:3, p. 294. An exploration of the contradictions involved in new technologies and the ways that these dilemmas affect women.

McDonald, Peter. "Gender Equity in Theories of Fertility Transition." *Population and Development Review.* September 2000. 26:3, p. 427. Low fertility in advanced countries, argues the author, is because women have achieved gender equality in the public sphere while still struggling with inequality in the private/family sphere.

McGee, Glenn. "Cloning, Sex, and New Kinds of Families." *The Journal of Sex Research.* August 2000, 37:3, p. 266. A positive look at the way that cloning might reshape the family.

Motluk, Alison. "Total Control?" *New Scientist.* December 2, 2000, 168:2267, p. 40. An interview with Roger Gosden, a fertility expert speaking about how technology is reshaping our ideas of conception and pregnancy.

Olagundoye, V.O. "The Value of Gonadrotrophin Releasing Hormone Analogue in an Intrauterine Insemination (IUI) Programme." *Journal of Obstetrics and Gynaecology.* March 2000, 20:2, p. 175. A look at the controversy surrounding gonadotrophin releasing hormone analogue (GnRHa).

Parker, Michael. "Public Deliberation and Private Choice in Genetics and Reproduction." *Journal of Medical Ethics.* June 2000, 26:3, p. 160. A question of what "patient-centeredness" means in a medical world in which genetic technology is available.

Pook, M. "A Validation Study of the Negative Association Between an Active Coping Style and Sperm Concentration." *Journal of Reproductive and Infant Psychology*. August 2000, 18:3, p. 249. A study exploring the hypothesis that men with an active coping style have a lower concentration of sperm.

Puddifoot, John. "Embodied Progress: A Cultural Account of Assisted Conception." *Social Science & Medicine*. June 2000, 50:11, p. 1696. Book review.

Raloff, Janet. "Prenatal Exposures Affect Sperm Later." *Science News*. November 4, 2000, 158: 19, p. 303. A 1979 industrial accident in Taiwan affected the fertility of young men who were in the wombs of women exposed to the toxins.

Sentker, Andreas. "Preimplantation Diagnosis Debate Rumbles on in Germany." *Lancet*. June 3, 2000, 355:9219, p. 1980. The German Medical Assembly has issued guidelines on preimplantation genetic diagnosis (PGD), which is so far not legal in Germany.

Shelton, Deborah L. "Pregnancy Rates Soaring in Older Moms." *American Medical News*. July 24, 2000, 43:27, p. 25. Postponing motherhood has become more desirable and less risky thanks to new career opportunities and advancements in ART.

Stephen, Elizabeth Hervey, and Anjani Chandra. "Use of Infertility Services in the United States: 1995." *Family Planning Perspectives*. May/June 2000, 32:3, p. 243. Women who have used infertility services are only a small minority of women with fertility problems; most women who do seek services receive noninvasive treatments.

Waiz, Nashid Kamal. "Role of Education in the Use of Contraception." *Lancet*, December 2000, vol. 356:51, p. S51. Education seems to help reduce the birth rate by increasing the number of women who use contraception.

Wang, J.X. "Body Mass and Probability of Pregnancy During Assisted Reproduction Treatment; Retrospective Study." *British Medical Journal*. November 25, 2000, 321:7272, p. 1,320. Both underweight and overweight women have some difficulties reproducing.

Westhoff, Carolyn. "Tubal Sterilization—Safe and Effective." *New England Journal of Medicine*. December 7, 2000, 343:23, p. 1,724. The continuing popularity of tubal sterilization in the United States shows how strongly women want to control their fertility.

Zhang, Jie. "Long-run Implications of Social Security Taxation for Growth and Fertility." *Southern Economic Journal*. January 2001, 67:3, p. 713. Social Security taxation affects fertility in a variety of ways.

Zweig, Franklin M. "With Reproductive Freedom and Distributive Justice for All: The Ethics of Genetic Manipulation." *American Scientist*. January/February 2001, 89:1, p. 77. Book review.

WEB SITES

Abortion Clinics On-Line. Available online. URL: http://www.gynpages. com. Downloaded March 13, 2001. A directory of more than 400 providers of abortions and other reproductive health care, with specific information about RU-486, late abortion, emergency contraception, and tubal ligation. The site features continually updated links to other sources of news and information, such as press releases from the FDA, articles on abortion rights, web sites featuring research on abortion, abortion-related news stories, and links to feminist and reproductive rights groups.

Advocates for Youth. Available online. URL: http://www.advocatesforyouth. org. Downloaded March 13, 2001. An organization dedicated to helping young people make responsible decisions about their sexual health. The web site provides a wide range of information about the United States and rest of the world.

Alan Guttmacher Institute. Available online. URL: http://www.agi-usa.org. Downloaded March 13, 2001. A research and policy institute devoted to expanding reproductive choice. The web site offers access to journal articles and reports on teen pregnancy, contraception, abortion, sexual behavior, law and public policy, and other topics, including sexually transmitted diseases and HIV.

American College of Obstetricians and Gynecologists (ACOG). Available online. URL: http://www.acog.org. Downloaded March 13, 2001. The web site for ACOG, a private, voluntary, nonprofit membership organization for professionals who provide health care for women. This is good source of information on fertility techniques and the profession's response to them.

American Collegians for Life. Available online. URL: http://www.ACLife. org. Downloaded March 13, 2001. A student-run nonprofit group dedicated to educating college students about abortion, infanticide, and euthanasia. The web site has information on college-based pro-life events.

American Life League. Available online. URL: http://www.all.org. Downloaded March 14, 2001. The nation's largest pro-life educational organization sponsors this web site, which provides information on abortion, assisted suicide, bioethics, birth control, cloning, end-of-life care, eugenics, and fetal research.

American Medical Women's Association (AMWA). Available online. URL: http://www.amwa-doc.org. Downloaded March 13, 2001. A pro-choice group for women doctors, whose web site provides information about health topics, links to other sites with reproductive health information, and information for medical students.

Annotated Bibliography

American Society for Reproductive Medicine (ASRM). Available online. URL: http://www.asrm.org. Downloaded March 13, 2001. The web site for ASRM, the voluntary, nonprofit membership organization for fertility specialists (formerly the American Fertility Society). The Patient Information Series of booklets available through this group can be a useful way of finding out new information on reproductive technology, explained in lay terms.

Americans United for Life (AUL). Available online. URL: http://www.unitedforlife.org. Downloaded March 14, 2001. A national public-interest law firm dedicated to abolishing abortion and euthanasia. Its online archive of news releases and its online forum are a useful way of reviewing key developments in the pro-life movement.

Association of American Physicians and Surgeons (AAPS). Available online. URL: http://www.aapsonline.org. Downloaded March 13, 2001. A nonpartisan medical association that also accepts medical students and patients, founded in 1943. Information about medical issues is available on its web site.

Association of Reproductive Health Professionals (ARHP). Available online. URL: http://www.arhp.org. Downloaded March 13, 2001. An interdisciplinary association of professionals involved in reproductive health services, education, research, or policy. The group publishes and/or sponsors a number of journals, newsletters, and other publications and offers educational materials available online.

Biblical American Resistance Front (BARF). Available online. URL: http://www.barf.org. Downloaded March 14, 2001. A resource for groups and individuals who oppose the influence of what it calls "Biblical America": the Religious Right and all those who see a particular reading of the Bible as the basis for governing American society. The web site features provocative articles about abortion as well as profiles and interviews of leading pro-life figures such as Dr. Bernard Nathanson.

Black Americans for Life. Available online. URL: http://www.NRLC.org/outreach/bal.html. Downloaded March 14, 2001. A pro-life organization that focuses on African Americans.

Campaign for Our Children, Inc. Available online. URL: http://www.cfoc.org. Downloaded March 14, 2001. An organization aimed at reducing teen pregnancy in Maryland, with news releases, facts, statistics, resources, research, and other information about teen pregnancy.

Catholic Alliance. Available online. URL: http://www.catholicvote.org. Downloaded March 14, 2001. A legislative group representing the Catholic perspective, particularly on abortion and reproductive rights issues.

Catholics for a Free Choice. Available online. URL: http://www.cath4choice. org. Downloaded March 14, 2001. A Catholic group that supports reproductive rights. Information and resources are available on the web site.

The Center for Bioethics and Human Dignity. Available online. URL: http://www.bioethix.org. Downloaded March 14, 2001. A division of the American Life League whose mission is to provide information for people and groups interested in reproductive technologies, as well as managed care, end-of-life treatment, genetic intervention, and euthanasia. This pro-life group offers a range of online resources, including links to other web sites, press releases on key issues, and links to mainstream news articles.

Center for Male Reproductive Medicine and Microsurgery. Available online. URL: http://www. maleinfertility.org. Downloaded March 13, 2001. This center, located at Cornell University, provides state-of-the-art treatment for infertile men, as well as conducting research and educational programs. Useful information on male infertility is available through their web site.

Center for Reproductive Law and Policy. Available online. URL: http:// www.crlp.org. Downloaded March 14, 2001. A pro-choice group whose goal is to support safe and healthy pregnancies; safe, accessible, and legal abortion; and other women's health issues. Its web site includes information on current hot topics, U.S. and international issues, press information, and the group's newsletter.

Centers for Disease Control and Prevention (CDC). Available online. URL: http://www.cdc.gov. Downloaded March 13, 2001. A useful site to find statistics on health issues, including a 1998 report on the effectiveness of ART: http://www.cdc.gov/ncchphp/drh/art98.

Contraceptive Research and Development Program (CONRAD). Available online. URL: http://www.conrad.org. Downloaded March 14, 2001. A group committed to finding better contraceptive methods, especially those that can be used worldwide. Based at Eastern Virginia Medical School, the organization produces a number of publications and makes contraceptive information available. Much of its information can be accessed online.

EMILY's List. Available online. URL: http://www.emilyslist.org. EMILY's List is a nationwide network of political donors dedicated to electing pro-choice Democratic women. Political information is available through the group's web site.

EngenderHealth. Available online. URL: http://www.engenderhealth.org. Downloaded March 14, 2001. A group that advocates for women's health issues internationally. The web site offers information on family planning, maternal/child health, men's health, postabortion care, infections, and sexuality and gender.

Ethics: Abortion. Available online. URL: http://ethics.acusd.edu/abortion. html. Downloaded March 14, 2001. This is one portion of a web site devoted to offering wide-ranging discussions on the ethics of various issues. This section, on abortion, includes a wide variety of resources, including links to court decisions, Gallup polls on abortion, Papal documents, web links, popular articles, and online articles. An extremely broad and useful look at the topic from many different perspectives.

Family Health International (FHI). Available online. URL: http://www. FHI.org. Downloaded March 14, 2001. A group dedicated to improving the well-being of international populations, offering information on family planning and HIV/AIDS. More than 1,500 full-text materials are available online, including FHI periodicals, working papers, reports, and training materials.

Family Research Council (FRC). Available online. URL: http://www.frc. org. Downloaded March 14, 2001. A multi-issue Religious Right group that takes an active nationwide role in advocating pro-life causes. The group's web site offers a wide variety of materials on many issues, including the national pro-life movement.

Feminists for Life of America. Available online. URL: http://www. feministsforlife.org. A group that calls itself "pro woman, pro life" and says that it is "continuing the tradition of Susan B. Anthony." Feminists for Life deals with a range of issues that bring together feminist concerns with a pro-life position. The group also opposes capital punishment, euthanasia and assisted suicide, and child abuse. Information about Feminists for Life's positions are available through its web site.

Ferre Institute. Available online. URL: http://www.ferre.org. Downloaded March 13, 2001. A nonprofit organization devoted to educational services, focusing on infertility, reproductive health, and the building of families; a newsletter, videotapes, and brochures are available.

Global Reproductive Health Forum: Research Library. Available online. URL: http://www.hsph.harvard.edu/Organizations/healthnet. A service provided by the Harvard School of Public Health, providing information on contraception methods and other related issues.

Health Finder. Available online. URL: http://www.healthfinder.gov. Downloaded March 14, 2001. A government-sponsored web site with information on a variety of health topics, as well as news, online journals, medical dictionaries, databases, libraries, and other resources.

International Council on Infertility Information Dissemination (INCIID). Available online. URL: http://www.inciid.org. Downloaded March 13, 2001. A nonprofit group that provides information on infertility and pregnancy loss, offering a great deal of information over the web.

JAMA Women's Health Contraception Information Center. Available online. URL: http://www.ama-assn.org/special/contra/contra.htm. Downloaded

March 14, 2001. A list of web links on contraception and reproductive rights, maintained by the *Journal of the American Medical Association (JAMA)*.

Kaiser Family Foundation. Available online. URL: http://www.kff.org. Downloaded March 14, 2001. Users who register with this site can get regular e-mail updates on reproductive health issues and other health-related topics.

Medem. Available online. URL: http://www.medem.com. A medical information service partly maintained by the American College of Obstetricians and Gynecologists, with a huge base of information on women's health and other medical issues.

Medical Students for Choice (MSFC). Available online. URL: http://www.ms4c.org. Downloaded March 14, 2001. A group that helps medical students improve education about reproductive health issues in U.S. medical schools.

National Abortion and Reproductive Rights Action League (NARAL). Available online. URL: http://www.naral.org. Downloaded March 14, 2001. The web site of the major U.S. abortion rights group; a rich source of information, with access to NARAL publications on reproductive rights issues nationwide.

National Campaign to Prevent Teen Pregnancy. Available online. URL: http://www.teenpregnancy.org. Downloaded March 14, 2001. A national group seeking to prevent teen pregnancy, whose web site offers facts and figures, tips for parents and teens, reading lists, the Campaign's publications, and other teen-related information.

National Coalition for Life and Peace. Available online. URL: http://www.prolifeinfo.org.nclp/. Downloaded March 14, 2001. A coalition of pro-life groups and individuals who oppose abortion-related violence, particularly the clinic-related violence that resulted in the deaths of abortion providers. The group also opposes web sites that might promote such violence. Information on the group and its position is available through its web site.

National Family Planning and Reproductive Health Association (NFPRHA). Available online. URL: http://www.nfprha.org. Downloaded March 14, 2001. A group working to assure access to voluntary family planning and reproductive health services. The web site includes fact sheets on teen pregnancy and other topics.

National Organization for Women (NOW). Available online. URL: http://www.now.org. Downloaded March 14, 2001. One of the best-established women's groups, and a strong supporter of reproductive rights. The web site offers news highlights, a forum, and other information.

National Organization on Adolescent Pregnancy, Parenting, and Prevention (NOAPPP). Available online. URL: http://www.noappp.org. Downloaded: March 14, 2001. A group that deals with teen pregnancy, parenting, and prevention, whose web site offers access to the group's newsletters on such topics as violence and teen pregnancy.

National Right to Life Organization. Available online. URL: http://www. nrlc.org. Downloaded March 14, 2001. The oldest, best-established right-to-life group, whose online site offers a daily commentary on pro-life issues, legislative updates, embryo research, and a range of current hot topics. Pro-life speeches by political figures and news releases can also be found at this site.

Not-2-Late.com: The Emergency Contraception Website. Available online. URL: http://www.ec.princeton.edu/. Downloaded March 14, 2001. A site with the latest and most detailed information available on emergency contraception, maintained by a Princeton University group and peer-reviewed by a panel of outside experts.

Office of Population Research. Available online. URL: http://www.opr. princeton.edu. Downloaded March 14, 2001. The oldest population research center in the United States, established in 1936 at Princeton University. Its web site offers a vast array of resources including a data archive and library, as well as information on gender, development, and emergency contraception.

Operation Save America. Available online. URL: http://www. operationsaveamerica.org. The group once known as Operation Rescue and famous for pioneering direct action against abortion clinics now has a new name and a broader focus: opposing gay rights and gay/lesbian marriage as well as trying to stop abortion.

Planned Parenthood. Available online. URL: http://www.plannedparenthood. org. Probably the single most useful source of information for those interested in reproductive rights and technology from a pro-choice perspective, as the site offers information about court decisions, contraception, and links to sites giving information about teen pregnancy and reproductive rights groups.

Population Council. Available online. URL: http://www.popcouncil.org. Downloaded March 14, 2001. This group's mission is to improve the reproductive health of current and future generations and to achieve a sustainable balance between people and resources. A wide range of national and international information is available through their web site.

Priests for Life. Available online. URL: http://www.priestsforlife.org. Downloaded March 14, 2001. A group whose mission is to inspire Catholic priests to take an active role in opposing abortion. The web site offers a chance to subscribe to a biweekly pro-life column by a priest as well as providing information about other pro-life groups.

Pro-Life Action League (PLAN). Available online. URL: http://www. prolifeaction.org. Downloaded March 14, 2001. A pro-life group based in Chicago, "dedicated to saving lives through activism and bringing the abortion issue to the public via the media." The group is headed by Joseph Scheidler, credited by many with helping to create pro-life direct action.

Pro-Life Alliance of Gays and Lesbians (PLAGAL). Available online. URL: http://www.plagal.org. Downloaded March 14, 2001. This group believes that gays, lesbians, and the unborn share a common oppression. Their web site offers newsletters, media releases, and brochures.

Religious Coalition for Reproductive Choice. Available online. URL: http://www.rcrc.org. Downloaded March 14, 2001. A group supporting reproductive choice from a religious perspective, claiming that mainstream America is both pro-faith and pro-choice. A range of information on news events, faith groups, and Black churches is available at this site, as well as sermons and prayers, pro-choice arguments, and discussions of religion and choice.

Reproductive Health Reproline Online. Available online. URL: http:// www.reproline.jhu.edu. Downloaded March 14, 2001. A web site that offers information on family planning, cervical cancer, and a range of reproductive health issues.

RESOLVE. Available online. URL: http://www.resolve.org. Downloaded March 13, 2001. A major national organization that offers counseling and education on infertility.

Roe No More Ministry. Available online. URL: http://www.roenomore.org. Downloaded March 14, 2001. The web site maintained by Norma McCorvey, the abortion rights activist who took the pseudonym "Roe" and helped bring the suit that resulted in *Roe v. Wade.* Later, McCorvey became disillusioned with feminism and reproductive rights and established her own ministry and web site to oppose abortion. The web site offers information on the "real story" behind *Roe v. Wade* and other facts about McCorvey, as well as access to a speakers' bureau and press information.

Sexuality Information and Education Council of the United States (SIECUS). Available online. URL: http://www.siecus.org. Downloaded March 14, 2001. This organization maintains the most comprehensive library of sex education materials in the world, and offers information and the chance to order publications online.

Ultimate Pro-Life Resource List. Available online. URL: http://www. prolifeinfo.org. Downloaded March 14, 2001. The most comprehensive listing of right-to-life resources on the Internet; however, since the site strongly opposes abortion-related violence, it does not include such groups in its listing. With that exception, the site has a huge range of pro-life groups, including national organizations, state groups, local organizations, college groups, Canadian organizations, international organizations, groups related to political parties, organizations that oppose euthanasia, health-related groups, abortion alternatives, postabortion counseling and information, and religious groups.

University Faculty for Life (UFL). Available online. URL: http://www2. franuniv.edu/ufl/home.html. Downloaded March 14, 2001. A group founded in 1989 to help pro-life faculty members. The web site offers a newsletter and other sources of information.

CHAPTER 8

ORGANIZATIONS

This chapter lists all of the major organizations concerning reproductive rights and technology. The groups have been divided into three categories: Pro-Choice, Pro-Life, and Scientific/Informational. There is a great deal of overlap in the kind of information that each group offers—for example, all three types of groups might offer a description of a certain type of abortion or statistics on teenagers' use of contraception. However, it seemed most useful to categorize the groups so that readers could readily identify the major purpose of each organization.

PRO-CHOICE GROUPS

Advocates for Youth
Suite 200
1025 Vermont Avenue, NW
Washington, DC 20005
Phone: (202) 347-5000
Fax: (202) 347-2263
E-mail: info@advocatesforyouth.
  org
URL: http://www.advocatesfor-
  youth.org.
An organization dedicated to help-
ing young people make responsible
decisions about their sexual health;
the group offers a wide range of in-

formation about the United States
and the rest of the world.

Alan Guttmacher Institute
120 Wall Street
New York, NY 10005
Phone: (212) 248-1111
Fax: (212) 248-1951
E-mail: info@agi-usa.org
  buyit@agi-usa.org
  mediaworks@agi-usa.org
120 Connecticut Avenue, NW
Suite 460
Washington, DC 20036
Phone: (202) 296-4012
Fax: (202) 223-5756
E-mail: policyinfo@agi-usa.org
URL: http://www.agi-usa.org

A research and policy institute devoted to expanding reproductive choice.

American Medical Women's Association (AMWA)
801 N. Fairfax Street
Suite 400
Alexandria, VA 22314
Phone: (703) 838-0500
Fax: (703) 549-3864
e-mail: info@amwa-doc.org
URL: http://www.amwa-doc.org.
A pro-choice group for women doctors, offering information about health topics, links to other sites with reproductive health information, and information for medical students.

Campaign for Our Children, Inc.
120 West Fayette Street
Suite 1200
Baltimore, MD 21201
Phone: (410) 576-9015
URL: http://www.cfoc.org.
An organization aimed at reducing teen pregnancy in Maryland, with news releases, facts, statistics, resources, research, and other information about teen pregnancy.

Catholics for a Free Choice
1436 U Street, NW
Suite 301
Washington, DC 20009-3997
Phone: (202) 986-6093
Fax: (202) 332-7995
URL: http://www.cath4choice.
  org

A Catholic group that supports reproductive rights and operates worldwide.

Center for Reproductive Law and Policy
120 Wall Street
New York, NY 10005
Phone: (917) 637-3600
Fax: (917) 647-4666
E-mail: info@clrp.org
1146 19th Street, NW
Washington, DC 20036
Phone: (202) 530-2975
Fax: (202) 530-2976
E-mail: info@crlp.org
URL: http://www.crlp.org
A pro-choice group that advocates for safe and healthy pregnancies; safe, accessible, and legal abortion; and other women's health issues. It provides information on current hot topics and U.S. and international issues.

EMILY's List
805 15th Street, NW
Suite 400
Washington, DC 20005
Phone: (202) 326-1400
URL: http://www.emilyslist.org
EMILY's List is a nationwide network of political donors dedicated to electing pro-choice Democratic women. Political information on reproductive rights is available.

EngenderHealth
440 Ninth Avenue,
Third Floor
New York, NY 10001

211

Phone: (212) 561-8000
Fax: (212) 561-8067
URL: http://www.
engenderhealth.org
A group that advocates for women's health issues internationally and provides information on family planning, maternal/child health, men's health, postabortion care, infections, and sexuality and gender.

Family Health International (FHI)
P.O. Box 13950
Research Triangle Park, NC 27709
Phone: (919) 544-7040
Fax: (919) 544-7261
URL: http://www.FHI.org
A group dedicated to improving the well-being of international populations, with information on family planning and HIV/AIDS, offering more than 1,500 full-text materials available online, including FHI periodicals, working papers, reports, and training materials.

Medical Students for Choice (MSFC)
2041 Bancroft Way
Suite 201
Berkeley, CA 94704
E-mail: msfc@ms4c.org
URL: http://www.ms4c.org
A group that helps medical students improve education about reproductive health issues in U.S. medical schools.

National Abortion and Reproductive Rights Action League (NARAL)
1156 15th Street
Suite 700
Washington, DC 20005
Phone: (202) 973-3000
Fax: (202) 973-3096
URL: http://www.naral.org
The major abortion rights groups in the United States; a rich source of information, offering many publications on reproductive rights issues nationwide.

National Family Planning and Reproductive Health Association (NFPRHA)
1627 K Street, NW
12th Floor
Washington, DC 20006
Phone: (202) 293-3114
Fax: (202) 293-1990
URL: http://www.nfprha.org
A group working to assure access to voluntary family planning and reproductive health services.

National Organization for Women (NOW)
733 15th Street, NW
Second Floor
Washington, DC 20005
Phone: (202) 628-8669
Fax: (202) 785-8576
E-mail: now@now.org
URL: http://www.now.org
One of the best-established women's groups and a strong supporter of reproductive rights.

212

Organizations

Planned Parenthood Federation of America
1 Oakbrook Terrace
#806
Oakbrook Terrace, IL 60181
Phone: (630) 627-9270
Fax: (630) 627-9549
1780 Massachusetts Avenue, NW
Washington, DC 20036
Phone: (202) 785-3351
Fax: (202) 293-4349
URL: http://www.plannedparenthood.org
The oldest and best-established reproductive rights group in the United States.

Religious Coalition for Reproductive Choice
1025 Vermont Avenue, NW
Suite 1130
Washington, DC 20005
Phone: (202) 628-7700
Fax: (202) 628-7716
E-mail: info@rcrc.org
URL: http://www.rcrc.org
A religious group that supports reproductive choice, claiming that mainstream America is both pro-faith and pro-choice.

Sexuality Information and Education Council of the United States (SIECUS)
130 W. 42nd Street
Suite 350
New York, NY 10036-7802
Phone: (212) 819-9770
Fax: (212) 819-9776
E-mail: siecus@siecus.org
URL: http://www.siecus.org
A group devoted to gathering and making available information about sexuality and sex education.

PRO-LIFE GROUPS

American Collegians for Life
P.O. Box 1112
Washington, DC 20013
Phone: (202) 737-1007
E-mail: acl@aclife.org
URL: http://www.ACLife.org
A student-run nonprofit group dedicated to educating college students about abortion, infanticide, and euthanasia.

American Life League
P.O. Box 1350
Stafford, VA 22333
Phone: (540) 659-4171
URL: http://www.all.org
The nation's largest pro-life educational organization, providing information on abortion, assisted suicide, bioethics, birth control, cloning, end-of-life care, eugenics, and fetal research.

Americans United for Life (AUL)
310 South Peoria Street
Suite 300
Chicago, IL 60607-3534
Phone: (312) 492-7234

Fax: (312) 492-7235
URL: http://www.unitedforlife.
  org
A national public-interest law firm
dedicated to abolishing abortion
and euthanasia.

Black Americans for Life
419 7th Street, NW
Suite 500
Washington, DC 20004
URL: http://www.NRLC.org/
  outreach/bal.html.
A pro-life organization that focuses
on African Americans.

Catholic Alliance
448 New Jersey Avenue, SE
Washington, DC 20003-4008
URL: http://www.catholicvote.
  org
A legislative group representing the
Catholic perspective, particularly on
abortion and reproductive rights.

The Center for Bioethics and
** Human Dignity**
2065 Half Day Road
Bannockburn, IL 60015
Phone: (847) 317-8180
Fax: (847) 317-8153
E-mail: cbhd@cbhd.org
URL: http://www.bioethix.org
A division of the American Life
League whose mission is to provide
information for people and groups
interested in reproductive tech-
nologies, as well as managed care,
end-of-life treatment, genetic in-
tervention, and euthanasia.

The Christian Broadcasting
** Network**
977 Centerville Turnpike
Virgina Beach, VA 23463
Phone: (757) 226-7000
Major multi-issue group that comes
out strongly against abortion and
other reproductive rights issues,
founded by Rev. Pat Robertson;
sponsors *The 700 Club TV Show*.

The Christian Coalition
1801 Sarah Drive
Suite L
Chesapeake, VA 23320
Phone: (804) 424-2630
Major Religious Right group that
takes on many issues, including
abortion and other reproductive
rights issues, headed by Ralph
Reed.

Family Research Council (FRC)
801 G Street, NW
Washington, DC 20001
Phone: (202) 393-2100
Fax: (202) 393-2134
Major Religious Right group that
deals with many family issues, including opposing abortion and
other reproductive choices, headed
by Gary Bauer.

Feminists for Life of America
733 15th Street, NW
Suite 110
Washington, DC 20005
Phone: (202) 737-FFLA
URL: http://www.
  feministsforlife.org

A group that calls itself "pro woman, pro life" and says that it is "continuing the tradition of Susan B. Anthony," Feminists for Life deals with a range of issues that bring together feminist concerns with a pro-life position. The group also opposes capital punishment, euthanasia and assisted suicide, and child abuse.

Focus on the Family
1-800-A-FAMILY
Religious Right group that sees opposing abortion and other reproductive rights as part of its pro-family agenda, headed by Dr. James Dobson.

Liberty Counsel
P.O. Box 540774
Orlando, FL 32854
Phone: (407) 875-2100
Fax: (407) 875-0220
E-mail: liberty@lc.org
URL: http://www.lc.org
The group founded by Reverend Jerry Falwell to be a nationwide nonprofit religious group dedicated to preserving religious freedom and to opposing such issues as gay rights and abortion that are seen to be contrary to biblical law.

National Coalition for Life and Peace
E-mail: right2life@aol.com
URL: http://www.prolifeinfo. org.nclp.
A coalition of pro-life groups and individuals who oppose abortion-related violence, particularly the clinic-related violence that resulted in the deaths of abortion providers. The group also opposes web sites that it sees as promoting such violence.

National Right to Life Committee
419 7th Street, NW
Suite 500
Washington, DC 20004
Phone: (202) 626-8800
E-mail: NRLC@nrlc.org
URL: http://www.nrlc.org
The oldest, best-established right-to-life group.

Operation Save America
URL: http://www. operationsaveamerica.org.
The group, once known as Operation Rescue and famous for pioneering direct action against abortion clinics, now has a new name and a broader focus: opposing gay rights and gay/lesbian marriage as well as trying to stop abortion.

Priests for Life
P.O. Box 141172
Staten Island, NY 10314
Phone: (888) PFL-3448, (718) 980-4400
Fax: (718) 980-6515
E-mail: mail@priestsforlife.org
URL: http://www.priestsforlife. org
A group dedicated to inspiring Catholic priests to take an active role in pro-life activism.

Pro-Life Action League (PLAN)
6160 N. Cicero Avenue
Suite 600
Chicago, IL 60646
Phone: (773) 777-2900
Fax: (773) 777-3061
URL: http://www.prolifeaction.
org
A pro-life group based in Chicago, "dedicated to saving lives through activism and bringing the abortion issue to the public via the media." The group is headed by Joseph Scheidler, credited by many with helping to create pro-life direct action.

Pro-Life Alliance of Gays and Lesbians (PLAGAL)
P.O. Box 33293
Washington, DC 20033
Phone: (202) 223-6697
Fax: (202) 265-9737
E-mail: PLAGALOne@aol.com
URL: http://www.plagal.org
A group that sees gays, lesbians, and the unborn as sharing a common oppression.

Roe No More Ministry
P.O. Box 550626
Dallas, TX 75355
Phone: (214) 343-1069
Fax: (214) 353-8006
URL: http://www.roenomore.org
The ministry begun by Norma Mc-Corvey, the former abortion rights activist who took the pseudonym "Roe" and helped bring the suit that resulted in *Roe v. Wade.* Later, McCorvey became disillusioned with feminism and reproductive rights and established this ministry to oppose abortion.

University Faculty for Life (UFL)
120 New North Building
Georgetown University
Washington, DC 20057
E-mail: richard.fehring@ marquette.edu
URL: http://www2.franuniv.edu/ ufl/home.html
A group founded in 1989 to help pro-life faculty members promote their point of view.

SCIENTIFIC INFORMATIONAL

American College of Obstetricians and Gynecologists (ACOG)
409 12th Street, SW
P.O. Box 96920
Washington, DC 20090-6920
URL: http://www.acog.org
A private, voluntary, nonprofit membership organization for professionals who provide health care for women.

American Society for Reproductive Medicine (ASRM)
1209 Montgomery Highway
Birmingham, AL 35216-2809
Phone: (205) 978-5000
Fax: (205) 978-5005
E-mail: asrm@asrm.org
URL: http://www.asrm.org

Formerly the American Fertility Society, a voluntary, nonprofit membership organization for fertility specialists.

Association of Reproductive Health Professionals (ARHP)
2401 Pennsylvania Avenue, NW
Suite 350
Washington, DC 20037-1718
Fax: (202) 466-3826
URL: http://www.arhp.org
An interdisciplinary association of professionals involved in reproductive health services, education, research, or policy. The group publishes or sponsors a number of journals, newsletters, and other publications, and makes educational materials available online.

Center for Male Reproductive Medicine and Microsurgery
The New York Hospital-Cornell Medical Center
525 East 68th Street
New York, NY 10021
Phone: (212) 746-8153
URL: http://www.maleinfertility. org
This center provides state-of-the-art treatment for infertile men, as well as conducting research and educational programs. Useful information on male infertility is available through their web site.

Contraceptive Research and Development Program (CONRAD)
Eastern Virginia Medical School
1611 North Kent Street

Suite 806
Arlington, VA 22209
Phone: (703) 524-4744
Fax: (703) 524-4770
E-mail: info@conrad.org
URL: http://www.conrad.org
A group committed to finding better contraceptive methods, especially those that can be used worldwide.

Ferre Institute
258 Genesee Street
Suite 302
Utica, NY 13502
Phone: (315) 724-4348
E-mail: Ferrelnf@aol.com
URL: http://www.members.aol. com/ferreinf/ferre.html
A nonprofit organization devoted to educational services, focusing on infertility, reproductive health, and the building of families; a newsletter, videotapes, and brochures are available.

International Council on Infertility Information Dissemination (INCIID)
P.O. Box 6836
Arlington, VA 22206
Phone: (703) 379-9178
E-mail: INCIIDinfo@inciid.org
URL: http://www.inciid.org
A nonprofit group that provides information on infertility and pregnancy loss, offering a great deal of information over the web.

Office of Population Research
Wallace Hall
Princeton University
Princeton, NJ 08544

Phone: (609) 258-4870
Fax: (609) 258-1039
URL: http://www.opr.princeton.
  edu
The oldest population research center in the United States, established
in 1936 at Princeton University.

Population Council
One Dag Hammarskjold Plaza
New York, NY 10017
Phone: (212) 339-0500
Fax: (212) 755-6052
E-mail: pubinfo@popcouncil.org
URL: http://www.popcouncil.
  org
This group's mission is to improve
the reproductive health of current
and future generations and to
achieve a sustainable balance between people and resources. A wide
range of national and international
information is available through
their web site.

Population Information
  Program (PIP)
111 Market Place, Suite 310
Baltimore, MD 21202-4024
Phone: (410) 659-6300
Fax: (410) 659-6266
E-mail: Poprepts@jhuccp.org
URL: http://www.jhuccp.org
A group that publishes the online
quarterly journal *Population Reports*,
sponsored by the Johns Hopkins
School of Hygiene and Public
Health. It also publishes *The Essen-
tials of Contraceptive Technology: A
Handbook for the Clinic Staff*. The
journal is supported by the United
States Agency for International De-
velopment (USAID).

PART III

APPENDIX

APPENDIX

ROE V. WADE, 410 U.S. 113 (1973)

JUSTICE HARRY BLACKMUN: This Texas federal appeal . . . present[s] constitutional challenges to state criminal abortion legislation. The Texas statutes under attack here are typical of those that have been in effect in many States for approximately a century . . .

We forthwith acknowledge our awareness of the sensitive and emotional nature of the abortion controversy, of the vigorous opposing views, even among physicians, and of the deep and seemingly absolute convictions that the subject inspires. One's philosophy, one's experiences, one's exposure to the raw edges of human existence, one's religious training, one's attitudes toward life and family and their values, and the moral standards one establishes and seeks to observe, are all likely to influence and to color one's thinking and conclusions about abortion.

. . . "[The Constitution] is made for people of fundamentally differing views, and the accident of our finding certain opinions natural and familiar or novel and even shocking ought not to conclude our judgment upon the question whether statutes embodying them conflict with the Constitution of the United States."

The Texas statutes that concern us here . . . make it a crime to "procure an abortion," . . . or to attempt one, except with respect to "an abortion procured or attempted by medical advice for the purpose of saving the life of the mother." Similar statutes are in existence in a majority of the States.

Texas first enacted a criminal abortion statute in 1854. This was soon modified [in 1857, 1866, 1879, and 1911] into language that has remained substantially unchanged to the present time. The final article in each of these compilations provided the same exception . . . for an abortion by "medical advice for the purpose of saving the life of the mother."

Jane Roe [the name is a pseudonym], a single woman who was residing in Dallas County, Texas, instituted this federal action in March 1970 against the District Attorney of the county. She sought a declaratory judgment [a conclusive, binding statement by the court] that the Texas criminal abortion statutes were unconstitutional . . . and an injunction [an order from the court] restraining [preventing] the defendant [the District Attorney] from enforcing the statutes.

Roe [claimed] that she was unmarried and pregnant; that she wished to terminate her pregnancy by an abortion "performed by a competent, licensed physician, under safe, clinical conditions"; that she was unable to get a "legal" abortion in Texas because her life did not appear to be threatened by the continuation of her pregnancy; and that she could not afford to travel to another jurisdiction in order to secure a legal abortion under safe conditions. She claimed that the Texas statutes were unconstitutionally vague and that they abridged her right of personal privacy, protected by the First, Fourth, Fifth, Ninth, and Fourteenth Amendments. By an amendment to her complaint Roe purported to sue "on behalf of herself and all other women" similarly situated.

. . . Despite the use of the pseudonym, no suggestion is made that Roe is a fictitious person. For purposes of her case, we accept as true, and as established, her existence; her pregnant state, as of the inception of her suit in March 1970 and as late as May 21 of that year when she filed an alias affidavit with the District Court; and her inability to obtain a legal abortion in Texas.

Viewing Roe's case as of the time of its filing and thereafter until as late as May, there can be little dispute that it then presented a case or controversy and that . . . she, as a pregnant single woman thwarted by the Texas criminal abortion laws, had [the legal right] to challenge those statutes . . .

[Wade] notes, however, that the record does not disclose that Roe was pregnant at the time of the District Court hearing on May 22, 1970, or on the following June 17 when the court's opinion and judgment were filed. And he suggests that Roe's case must now be moot [no longer in controversy] because she . . . [is] no longer subject to any 1970 pregnancy.

The usual rule in federal cases is that an actual controversy must exist at stages of appellate . . . review, and not simply at the date the action is initiated.

But when, as here, pregnancy is a significant fact in the litigation, the normal 266-day human gestation period is so short that the pregnancy will come to term before the usual appellate process is complete. If that termination makes a case moot, pregnancy litigation seldom will survive much beyond the trial stage, and appellate review will be effectively denied. Our law should not be that rigid. Pregnancy often comes more than once to the same woman, and in the general population, if man is to survive, it will always be with us. Pregnancy provides a classic justification for a conclusion of nonmootness. It truly could be "capable of repetition, yet evading review."

We, therefore, agree with the District Court that Jane Roe had [the right] to undertake this litigation, that she presented a justiciable controversy, and that the termination of her 1970 pregnancy has not rendered her case moot.

. . . The principal thrust of appellant's attack on the Texas statutes is that they improperly invade a right, said to be possessed by the pregnant woman, to choose to terminate her pregnancy. [Roe claims] this right in the concept of personal "liberty" embodied in the Fourteenth Amendment's Due Process Clause; or in personal, marital, familial, and sexual privacy said to be protected by the Bill of Rights or its penumbras; or among those rights reserved to the people by the Ninth Amendment. Before addressing this claim, we feel it desirable briefly to survey, in several aspects, the history of abortion, for such insight as that history may afford us, and then to examine the state purposes and interests behind the criminal abortion laws.

It perhaps is not generally appreciated that the restrictive criminal abortion laws in effect in a majority of States today are of relatively recent vintage. Those laws, generally proscribing [prohibiting] abortion or its attempt at any time during pregnancy except when necessary to preserve the pregnant woman's life, are not of ancient or even of common-law origin. Instead, they derive from statutory [legislative] changes effected, for the most part, in the latter half of the 19th century.

1. Ancient attitudes. These are not capable of precise determination. We are told that at the time of the Persian Empire abortifacients were known and that criminal abortions were severely punished. We are also told, however, that abortion was practiced in Greek times as well as in the Roman Era, and that "it was resorted to without scruple." The Ephesian, Soranos, often described as the greatest of the ancient gynecologists, appears to have been generally opposed to Rome's prevailing free-abortion practices. He found it necessary to think first of the life of the mother, and he resorted to abortion when, upon this standard, he felt the procedure advisable. Greek and Roman law afforded little protection to the unborn. If abortion was prosecuted in some places, it seems to have been based on a concept of a violation of the father's right to his offspring. Ancient religion did not bar abortion.

2. The Hippocratic Oath. What then of the famous Oath that has stood so long as the ethical guide of the medical profession and that bears the name of the great Greek, who has been described as the Father of Medicine, the "wisest and the greatest practitioner of his art," and the "most important and most complete medical personality of antiquity," who dominated the medical schools of his time, and who typified the sum of the medical

knowledge of the past? The Oath varies somewhat according to the particular translation, but in any translation the content is clear: "I will give no deadly medicine to anyone if asked, nor suggest any such counsel; and in like manner I will not give to a woman a pessary to produce abortion," or "I will neither give a deadly drug to anybody if asked for it, nor will I make a suggestion to this effect. Similarly, I will not give to a woman an abortive remedy."

Although the Oath is not mentioned in any of the principal briefs in this case . . . , it represents the apex of the development of strict ethical concepts in medicine, and its influence endures to this day. Why did not the authority of Hippocrates dissuade abortion practice in his time and that of Rome? The late Dr. Edelstein provides us with a theory: The Oath was not uncontested even in Hippocrates' day; only the Pythagorean school of philosophers frowned upon the related act of suicide. Most Greek thinkers, on the other hand, commended abortion, at least prior to viability. For the Pythagoreans, however, it was a matter of dogma. For them the embryo was animate from the moment of conception, and abortion meant destruction of a living being. The abortion clause of the Oath, therefore, "echoes Pythagorean doctrines," and "[i]n no other stratum of Greek opinion were such views held or proposed in the same spirit of uncompromising austerity."

Dr. Edelstein then concludes that the Oath originated in a group representing only a small segment of Greek opinion and that it certainly was not accepted by all ancient physicians. He points out that medical writings down to Galen (A.D. 130-200) "give evidence of the violation of almost every one of its injunctions." But with the end of antiquity a decided change took place. Resistance against suicide and against abortion became common. The Oath came to be popular. The emerging teachings of Christianity were in agreement with the Pythagorean ethic. The Oath "became the nucleus of all medical ethics" and "was applauded as the embodiment of truth." Thus, suggests Dr. Edelstein, it is "a Pythagorean manifesto and not the expression of an absolute standard of medical conduct."

This, it seems to us, is a satisfactory and acceptable explanation of the Hippocratic Oath's apparent rigidity. It enables us to understand, in historical context, a long-accepted and revered statement of medical ethics.

3. The common law. It is undisputed that at common law [court decisions], abortion performed *before* "quickening"—the first recognizable movement of the fetus in utero, appearing usually from the 16th to the 18th week of pregnancy—was not an indictable offense. The absence of a common-law crime for pre-quickening abortion appears to have developed from a confluence of earlier philosophical, theological, and civil and canon law concepts of when life begins. These disciplines variously approached the question in terms of the point at which the embryo or fetus became

"formed" or recognizably human, or in terms of when a "person" came into being, that is, infused with a "soul" or "animated." A loose consensus evolved in early English law that these events occurred at some point between conception and live birth. This was "mediate animation." Although Christian theology and the canon law came to fix the point of animation at 40 days for a male and 80 days for a female, a view that persisted until the 19th century, there was otherwise little agreement about the precise time of formation or animation. There was agreement, however, that prior to this point the fetus was to be regarded as part of the mother, and its destruction, therefore, was not homicide. Due to continued uncertainty about the precise time when animation occurred, to the lack of any empirical basis for the 40-80-day view, and perhaps to Aquinas' definition of movement as one of the two first principles of life, Bracton focused upon quickening as the critical point. The significance of quickening was echoed by later common-law scholars and found its way into the received [accepted] common law in this country.

Whether abortion of a *quick* fetus was a felony at common law, or even a lesser crime, is still disputed. Bracton, writing early in the 13th century, thought it homicide. But the later and predominant view, following the great common-law scholars, has been that it was, at most, a lesser offense. In a frequently cited passage, Coke took the position that abortion of a woman "quick with childe" is "a great misprision [an undefined crime], and no murder." Blackstone followed, saying that while abortion after quickening had once been considered manslaughter (though not murder), "modern law" took a less severe view. A recent review of the common-law precedents argues, however, that those precedents contradict Coke and that even post-quickening abortion was never established as a common-law crime. This is of some importance because while most American courts ruled, in holding [actual decision] or dictum [observations made in the decision], that abortion of an unquickened fetus was not criminal under their received common law, others followed Coke in stating that abortion of a quick fetus was a "misprision," a term they translated to mean "misdemeanor." That their reliance on Coke on this aspect of the law was uncritical and, apparently in all the reported cases, dictum (due probably to the paucity of common-law prosecutions for post-quickening abortion), makes it now appear doubtful that abortion was ever firmly established as a common-law crime even with respect to the destruction of a quick fetus.

4. The English statutory law. England's first criminal abortion statute, Lord Ellenborough's Act, came in 1803. It made abortion of a quick fetus . . . a capital crime, but . . . it provided lesser penalties for the felony of abortion before quickening, and thus preserved the "quickening" distinction. This contrast was continued in the general revision of 1828. It disappeared,

however, together with the death penalty, in 1837, and did not reappear in the Offenses Against the Person Act of 1861 that formed the core of English anti-abortion law until the liberalizing reforms of 1967. In 1929, the Infant Life (Preservation) Act came into being. Its emphasis was upon the destruction of "the life of a child capable of being born alive." It made a willful act performed with the necessary intent a felony. It contained a proviso that one was not to be found guilty of the offense "unless it is proved that the act which caused the death of the child was not done in good faith for the purpose only of preserving the life of the mother."

A seemingly notable development in the English law was the case of *Rex v. Bourne.* This case apparently answered in the affirmative the question whether an abortion necessary to preserve the life of the pregnant woman was excepted from the criminal penalties of the 1861 Act. In his instructions to the jury, Judge Macnaghten referred to the 1929 Act, and observed that that Act related to "the case where a child is killed by a wilful act at the time when it is being delivered in the ordinary course of nature." He concluded that the 1861 Act's use of the word "unlawfully," imported the same meaning expressed by the specific proviso in the 1929 Act, even though there was no mention of preserving the mother's life in the 1861 Act. He then construed the phrase "preserving the life of the mother" broadly, that is, "in a reasonable sense," to include a serious and permanent threat to the mother's *health*, and instructed the jury to acquit Dr. Bourne if it found he had acted in a good-faith belief that the abortion was necessary for this purpose. The jury did acquit.

Recently, Parliament enacted a new abortion law. This is the Abortion Act of 1967. The Act permits a licensed physician to perform an abortion where two other licensed physicians agree (a) "that the continuance of the pregnancy would involve risk to the life of the pregnant woman, or of injury to the physical or mental health of the pregnant woman or any existing children of her family, greater than if the pregnancy were terminated," or (b) "that there is a substantial risk that if the child were born it would suffer from such physical or mental abnormalities as to be seriously handicapped." The Act also provides that, in making this determination, "account may be taken of the pregnant woman's actual or reasonably foreseeable environment." It also permits a physician, without the concurrence of others, to terminate a pregnancy where he is of the good-faith opinion that the abortion "is immediately necessary to save the life or to prevent grave permanent injury to the physical or mental health of the pregnant woman."

5. The American law. In this country, the law in effect in all but a few States until mid-19th century was the preexisting English common law. Connecticut, the first State to enact abortion legislation, adopted in 1821 that part of Lord Ellenborough's Act that related to a woman "quick with

child." The death penalty was not imposed. Abortion before quickening was made a crime in that State only in 1860. In 1828, New York enacted legislation that, in two respects, was to serve as a model for early antiabortion statutes. First, while barring destruction of an unquickened fetus as well as a quick fetus, it made the former only a misdemeanor, but the latter second-degree manslaughter. Second, it incorporated a concept of therapeutic abortion by providing that an abortion was excused if it "shall have been necessary to preserve the life of such mother, or shall have been advised by two physicians to be necessary for such purpose." By 1840, when Texas had received the common law, only eight American States had statutes dealing with abortion. It was not until after the War Between the States that legislation began generally to replace the common law. Most of these initial statutes dealt severely with abortion after quickening but were lenient with it before quickening. Most punished attempts equally with completed abortions. While many statutes included the exception for an abortion thought by one or more physicians to be necessary to save the mother's life, that provision soon disappeared and the typical law required that the procedure actually be necessary for that purpose.

Gradually, in the middle and late 19th century the quickening distinction disappeared from the statutory law of most States and the degree of the offense and the penalties were increased. By the end of the 1950's, a large majority of the jurisdictions banned abortion, however and whenever performed, unless done to save or preserve the life of the mother. The exceptions, Alabama and the District of Columbia, permitted abortion to preserve the mother's health. Three States [Massachusetts, New Jersey, and Pennsylvania] permitted abortions that were not "unlawfully" performed or that were not "without lawful justification," leaving interpretation of those standards to the courts. In the past several years, however, a trend toward liberalization of abortion statutes has resulted in adoption, by about one-third of the States, of less stringent laws, most of them patterned after the ALI [American Law Institute]'s Model Penal Code . . .

It is thus apparent that at common law, at the time of the adoption of our Constitution, and throughout the major portion of the 19th century, abortion was viewed with less disfavor than under most American statutes currently in effect. Phrasing it another way, a woman enjoyed a substantially broader right to terminate a pregnancy than she does in most States today. At least with respect to the early stage of pregnancy, and very possibly without such a limitation, the opportunity to make this choice was present in this country well into the 19th century. Even later, the law continued for some time to treat less punitively an abortion procured in early pregnancy.

6. The position of the American Medical Association. The anti-abortion mood prevalent in this country in the late 19th century was shared by the

medical profession. Indeed, the attitude of the profession may have played a significant role in the enactment of stringent criminal abortion legislation during that period.

An AMA Committee on Criminal Abortion was appointed in May 1857. It presented its report to the Twelfth Annual Meeting. That report observed that the Committee had been appointed to investigate criminal abortion "with a view to its general suppression." It deplored abortion and its frequency and it listed three causes of "this general demoralization":

"The first of these causes is a wide-spread popular ignorance of the true character of the crime—a belief, even among mothers themselves, that the foetus is not alive till after the period of quickening.

"The second of the agents alluded to is the fact that the profession themselves are frequently supposed careless of foetal life . . .

"The third reason of the frightful extent of this crime is found in the grave defects of our laws, both common and statute, as regards the independent and actual existence of the child before birth, as living being. These errors, which are sufficient in most instances to prevent conviction, are based, and only based, upon mistaken and exploded medical dogmas. With strange inconsistency, the law fully acknowledges the foetus in utero and its inherent rights, for civil purposes; while personally and as criminally affected, it fails to recognize it, and to its life as yet denies all protection."

The Committee then offered, and the Association adopted, resolutions protesting "against such unwarrantable destruction of human life," calling upon state legislatures to revise their abortion laws, and requesting the cooperation of state medical societies "in pressing the subject."

In 1871 a long and vivid report was submitted by the Committee on Criminal Abortion. It ended with the observation, "We had to deal with human life. In a matter of less importance we could entertain no compromise. An honest judge on the bench would call things by their proper names. We could do not less." It proferred resolutions, adopted by the Association, recommending, among other things, that it "be unlawful and unprofessional for any physician to induce abortion or premature labor, without the concurrent opinion of at least one respectable consulting physician, and then always with a view to the safety of the child – if that be possible," and calling "the attention of the clergy of all denominations to the perverted views of mortality entertained by a large class of females—aye, and men also, on this important question."

Except for periodic condemnation of the criminal abortionist, no further formal AMA action took place until 1967. In that year, the Committee on Human Reproduction urged the adoption of a stated policy of opposition to induced abortion, except when there is "documented medical evidence" of a threat to the health or life of the mother, or that the child "may be born with incapacitating physical deformity or mental deficiency," or that a pregnancy "resulting from legally established statutory or forcible rape or incest may constitute a threat to the mental or physical health of the patient," and two other physicians "chosen because of their recognized professional competence have examined the patient and have concurred in writing," and the procedure "is performed in a hospital accredited by the Joint Commission on Accreditation of Hospitals." The providing of medical information by physicians to state legislatures in their consideration of legislation regarding therapeutic abortion was "to be considered consistent with the principles of ethics of the American Medical Association." This recommendation was adopted by the House of Delegates.

In 1970, after the introduction of a variety of proposed resolutions, and of a report from its Board of Trustees, a reference committee noted "polarization of the medical profession on this controversial issue"; division among those who had testified; a difference of opinion among AMA councils and committees; "the remarkable shift in testimony" in six months, felt to be influenced "by the rapid changes in state laws and by the judicial decisions which tend to make abortion more freely available"; and a feeling "that this trend will continue." On June 25, 1970, the House of Delegates adopted preambles and most of the resolutions proposed by the reference committee. The preambles emphasized "the best interests of the patient," "sound clinical judgment," and "informed patient consent," in contrast to "mere acquiescence to the patient's demand." The resolutions asserted that abortion is a medical procedure that should be performed by a licensed physician in an accredited hospital only after consultation with two other physicians and in conformity with state law, and that no party to the procedure should be required to violate personally held moral principles. The AMA Judicial Council rendered a complementary opinion.

7. The position of the American Public Health Association. In October 1970, the Executive Board of the APHA adopted Standards for Abortion Services. These were five in number:

"a. Rapid and simple abortion referral must be readily available through state and local public health departments, medical societies, or other nonprofit organizations.

"b. An important function of counseling should be to simplify and expedite the provision of abortion services; it should not delay the obtaining of these services.

"c. Psychiatric consultation should not be mandatory. As in the case of other specialized medical services, psychiatric consultation should be sought for definite indications and not on a routine basis.

"d. A wide range of individuals from appropriately trained, sympathetic volunteers to highly skilled physicians may qualify as abortion counselors.

"e. Contraception and/or sterilization should be discussed with each abortion patient."

Among factors pertinent to life and health risks associated with abortion were three that "are recognized as important":

"a. the skill of the physician,

"b. the environment in which the abortion is performed, and above all

"c. the duration of pregnancy, as determined by uterine size and confirmed by menstrual history."

It was said that "a well-equipped hospital" offers more protection "to cope with unforeseen difficulties than an office or clinic without such resources. . . . The factor of gestational age is of overriding importance." Thus, it was recommended that abortions in the second trimester and early abortions in the presence of existing medical complications be performed in hospitals as in-patient procedures. For pregnancies in the first trimester, abortion in the hospital with or without overnight stay "is probably the safest practice." An abortion in an extramural facility, however, is an acceptable alternative "provided arrangements exist in advance to admit patients promptly if unforeseen complications develop." Standards for an abortion facility were listed. It was said that at present abortions should be performed by physicians or osteopaths who are licensed to practice and who have "adequate training."

8. The position of the American Bar Association. At its meeting in February 1972 the ABA House of Delegates approved, with 17 opposing votes, the Uniform Abortion Act that had been drafted and approved the preceding August by the Conference of Commissioners on Uniform State Laws . . .

Three reasons have been advanced to explain historically the enactment of criminal abortion laws in the 19th century and to justify their continued existence.

It has been argued occasionally that these laws were the product of a Victorian social concern to discourage illicit sexual condut. Texas, however, does not advance this justification in the present case, and it appears that no court or commentator has taken the argument seriously. The appellants and amici [friends of the court] contend, moreover, that this is not a proper state purpose at all and suggest that, if it were, the Texas statutes are overbroad in protecting it since the law fails to distinguish between married and unwed mothers.

A second reason is concerned with abortion as a medical procedure. When most criminal abortion laws were first enacted, the procedure was a hazardous one for the woman. This was particularly true prior to the development of antisepsis. Antiseptic techniques, of course, were based on discoveries by Lister, Pasteur, and others first announced in 1867, but were not generally accepted and employed until about the turn of the century. Abortion mortality was high. Even after 1900, and perhaps until as late as the development of antibiotics in the 1940's, standard modern techniques such as dilation and curettage were not nearly so safe as they are today. Thus, it has been argued that a State's real concern in enacting a criminal abortion law was to protect the pregnant woman, that is, to restrain her from submitting to a procedure that placed her life in serious jeopardy.

Modern medical techniques have altered this situation. [Roe] . . . refer[s] to medical data indicating that abortion in early pregnancy, that is, prior to the end of the first trimester, although not without its risk, is now relatively safe. Mortality rates for women undergoing early abortions, where the procedure is legal, appear to be as low as or lower than the rates for normal childbirth. Consequently, any interest of the State in protecting the woman from an inherently hazardous procedure, except when it would be equally dangerous for her to forgo it, has largely disappeared. Of course, important state interests in the areas of health and medical standards do remain. The State has a legitimate interest in seeing to it that abortion, like any other medical procedure, is performed under circumstances that insure maximum safety for the patient. This interest obviously extends at least to the performing physician and his staff, to the facilities involved, to the availability of after-care, and to adequate provision for any complication or emergency that might arise. The prevalence of high mortality rates at illegal "abortion mills" strengthens, rather than weakens, the State's interest in regulating the conditions under which abortions are performed. Moreover, the risk to the woman increases as her pregnancy continues. Thus, the State retains a definite interest in protecting the woman's own health and safety when an abortion is proposed at a late stage of pregnancy.

The third reason is the State's interest—some phrase it in terms of duty—in protecting prenatal life. Some of the argument for this justification rests on the theory that a new human life is present from the moment of conception. The State's interest and general obligation to protect life then extends, it is argued, to prenatal life. Only when the life of the pregnant mother herself is at stake, balanced against the life she carries within her, should the interest of the embryo or fetus not prevail. Logically, of course, a legitimate state interest in this area need not stand or fall on acceptance of the belief that life begins at conception or at some other point prior to live birth. In assessing the State's interest, recognition may be given to the less rigid claim that as long as at least *potential* life is involved, the State may assert interests beyond the protection of the pregnant woman alone.

Parties challenging state abortion laws have sharply disputed in some courts the contention that a purpose of these laws, when enacted, was to protect prenatal life. Pointing to the absence of legislative history to support the contention, they claim that most state laws were designed solely to protect the woman. Because medical advances have lessened this concern, at least with respect to abortion in early pregnancy, they argue that with respect to such abortions the laws can no longer be justified by any state interest. There is some scholarly support for this view of original purpose. The few state courts called upon to interpret their laws in the late 19th and early 20th centuries did focus on the State's interest in protecting the woman's health rather than in preserving the embryo and fetus. Proponents of this view point out that in many States, including Texas, by statute or judicial interpretation, the pregnant woman herself could not be prosecuted for self-abortion or for cooperating in an abortion performed upon her by another. They claim that adoption of the "quickening" distinction through received common law and state statutes tacitly recognizes the greater health hazards inherent in late abortion and impliedly repudiates the theory that life begins at conception.

It is with these interests, and the weight to be attached to them, that this case is concerned.

The Constitution does not explicitly mention any right of privacy. In a line of decisions, however, going back perhaps as far as *Union Pacific R. Co. v. Botsford*, the Court has recognized that a right of personal privacy, or a guarantee of certain areas or zones of privacy, does exist under the Constitution. In varying contexts, the Court or individual Justices have, indeed, found at least the roots of that right in the First Amendment; in the Fourth and Fifth Amendments; in the penumbras of the Bill of Rights; in the Ninth Amendment; or in the concept of liberty guaranteed by the first section of the Fourteenth Amendment. . . . [O]nly personal rights that can be deemed "fundamental" or "implicit in the concept of ordered liberty" are included in this guarantee of personal privacy. . . . [T]he right has some extension to activities relating to marriage; procreation; contraception; family relationships; and child rearing and education.

This right of privacy, whether it be founded in the Fourteenth Amendment's concept of personal liberty and restrictions upon state action, as we feel it is, or, as the District Court determined, in the Ninth Amendment's reservation of rights to the people, is broad enough to encompass a woman's decision whether or not to terminate her pregnancy. The detriment that the State would impose upon the pregnant woman by denying this choice altogether is apparent. Specific and direct harm medically diagnosable even in early pregnancy may be involved. Maternity, or additional offspring, may force upon the woman a distressful life and future. Psychological harm may be imminent. Mental and physical health may be taxed by child care. There is also the distress, for all concerned, associated with the unwanted child, and there is the problem of bringing a child into a family already unable, psychologically and otherwise, to care for it. In other cases, as in this one, the additional difficulties and continuing stigma of unwed motherhood may be involved. All these are factors the woman and her responsible physician necessarily will consider in consultation.

On the basis of elements such as these, [Roe] argue[s] that the woman's right is absolute and that she is entitled to terminate her pregnancy at whatever time, in whatever way, and for whatever reason she alone chooses. With this we do not agree. [Roe]'s arguments that Texas either has no valid interest at all in regulating the abortion decision, or no interest strong enough to support any limitation upon the woman's sole determination, are unpersuasive. The Court's decisions recognizing a right of privacy also acknowledge that some state regulation in areas protected by that right is appropriate. As noted above, a State may properly assert important interests in safeguarding health, in maintaining medical standards, and in protecting potential life. At some point in pregnancy, these respective interests become sufficiently compelling to sustain regulation of the factors that govern the abortion decision. The privacy right involved, therefore, cannot be said to be absolute. In fact, it is not clear to us that the claim . . . that one has an unlimited right to do with one's body as one pleases bears a close relationship to the right of privacy previously articulated in the Court's decisions. The Court has refused to recognize an unlimited right of this kind in the past.

We, therefore, conclude that the right of personal privacy includes the abortion decision, but that this right is not unqualified and must be considered against important state interests in regulation.

We note that those federal and state courts that have recently considered abortion law challenges have reached the same conclusion. A majority, in addition to the District Court in the present case, have held state law unconstitutional, at least in part, because of vagueness or because of overbreadth and abridgment of rights.

Others have sustained state statutes.

Although the results are divided, most of these courts have agreed that the right of privacy, however based, is broad enough to cover the abortion decision; that the right, nonetheless, is not absolute and is subject to some limitations; and that at some point the state interests as to protection of health, medical standards, and prenatal life, become dominant. We agree with this approach.

Where certain "fundamental rights" are involved, the Court has held that regulation limiting these rights may be justified only by a "compelling state interest," and that legislative enactments must be narrowly drawn to express only the legitimate state interests at stake.

In the recent abortion cases . . . courts have recognized these principles. Those striking down state laws have generally scrutinized the State's interests in protecting health and potential life, and have concluded that neither interest justified broad limitations on the reasons for which a physician and his pregnant patient might decide that she should have an abortion in the early stages of pregnancy. Courts sustaining [letting stand] state laws have held that the State's determinations to protect health or prenatal life are dominant and constitutionally justifiable.

The District Court held that [Wade] failed to meet his burden of demonstrating that the Texas statute's infringement upon Roe's rights was necessary to support a compelling state interest, and that, although [Wade] presented "several compelling justifications for state presence in the area of abortions," the statutes outstripped these justifications and swept "far beyond any areas of compelling state interest." [Roe] and [Wade] both contest that holding.

[Roe], as has been indicated, claims an absolute right that bars any state imposition of criminal penalties in the area. [Wade] argues that the State's determination to recognize and protect prenatal life from and after conception constitutes a compelling state interest. As noted above, we do not agree fully with either formulation.

A. [Wade] and certain amici argue that the fetus is a "person" within the language and meaning of the Fourteenth Amendment. In support of this, they outline at length and in detail the well-known facts of fetal development. If this suggestion of personhood is established, [Roe]'s case, of course, collapses, for the fetus' right to life is then guaranteed specifically by the Amendment. [Roe] conceded as much on reargument. On the other hand, [Wade] conceded on reargument that no case could be cited that holds that a fetus is a person within the meaning of the Fourteenth Amendment.

The Constitution does not define "person" in so many words. Section 1 of the Fourteenth Amendment contains three references to "person." The first, in defining "citizens," speaks of "persons born or naturalized in the United States." The word also appears both in the Due Process Clause and in the Equal Protection Clause. "Person" is used in other places in the Constitution: in the listing of qualifications for Representatives and Senators; in the Apportionment Clause; in the Migration and Importation provision; in the Emolument Clause; in the Electors provisions; in the provision outlining qualifications for the office of President; in the Extradition provisions; and in the Fifth, Twelfth, and Twenty-second Amendments, as well as in [Sections] 2 and 3 of the Fourteenth Amendment. But in nearly all these instances, the use of the word is such that it has application only postnatally. None indicates, with any assurance, that it has any possible pre-natal application.

All this, together with our observation that throughout the major portion of the 19th century prevailing legal abortion practices were far freer than they are today, persuades us that the word "person," as used in the Fourteenth Amendment, does not include the unborn. This is in accord with the results reached in those few cases where the issue has been squarely presented. Indeed, our decision in *United States v. Vuitch* inferentially is to the same effect, for we there would not have indulged in statutory interpretation favorable to abortion in specified circumstances if the necessary consequence was the termination of life entitled to Fourteenth Amendment protection.

This conclusion, however, does not of itself fully answer the contentions raised by Texas, and we pass on to other considerations.

B. The pregnant woman cannot be isolated in her privacy. She carries an embryo and, later, a fetus, if one accepts the medical definitions of the developing young in the human uterus. The situation therefore is inherently different from marital intimacy, or bedroom possession of obscene material, or marriage, or procreation, or education. . . . As we have intimated above, it is reasonable and appropriate for a State to decide that at some point in time another interest, that of health of the mother or that of potential human life, becomes significantly involved. The woman's privacy is no longer sole and any right of privacy she processes must be measured accordingly.

Texas urges that, apart from the Fourteenth Amendment, life begins at conception and is present throughout pregnancy, and that, therefore, the State has a compelling interest in protecting that life from and after conception. We need not resolve the difficult question of when life begins. When those trained in the respective disciplines of medicine, philosophy, and theology are unable to arrive at any consensus, the judiciary, at this point in the development of man's knowledge, is not in a position to speculate as to the answer.

It should be sufficient to note briefly the wide divergence of thinking on this most sensitive and difficult question. There has always been strong support for the view that life does not begin until live birth. This was the belief of the Stoics. It appears to be the predominant, though not the unanimous, attitude of the Jewish faith. It may be taken to represent also the position of a large segment of the Protestant community, insofar as that can be ascertained; organized groups that have taken a formal position on the abortion issue have generally regarded abortion as a matter for the conscience of the individual and her family. As we have noted, the common law found greater significance in quickening. Physicians and their scientific colleagues have regarded that event with less interest and have tended to focus either upon conception, upon live birth, or upon the interim point at which the fetus becomes "viable," that is, potentially able to live outside the mother's womb, albeit with artificial aid. Viability is usually placed at about seven months (28 weeks) but may occur earlier, even at 24 weeks. The Aristotelian theory of "mediate animation," that held sway throughout the Middle Ages and the Renaissance in Europe, continued to be official Roman Catholic dogma until the 19th century, despite opposition to this "ensoulment" theory from those in the Church who would recognize the existence of life from the moment of conception. The latter is now, of course, the official belief of the Catholic Church. As one of the briefs amicus discloses, this is a view strongly held by many non-Catholics as well, and by many physicians. Substantial problems for precise definition of this view are posed, however, by new embryological data that purport to indicate that conception is a "process" over time, rather than an event, and by new medical techniques such as menstrual extraction, the "morning-after" pill, implantation of embryos, artificial insemination, and even artificial wombs.

In areas other than criminal abortion, the law has been reluctant to endorse any theory that life, as we recognize it, begins before live birth or to accord legal rights to the unborn except in narrowly defined situations and except when the rights are contingent upon live birth. For example, the traditional rule of tort law denied recovery for prenatal injuries even though the child was born alive. That rule has been changed in almost every jurisdiction. In most States, recovery is said to be permitted only if the fetus was viable, or at least quick, when the injuries were sustained, though few courts have squarely so held. In a recent development, generally opposed by the commentators, some States permit the parents of a stillborn child to maintain an action for wrongful death because of prenatal injuries. Such an action, however, would appear to be one to vindicate the parents' interest and is thus consistent with the view that the fetus, at most, represents only the potentiality of life. Similarly, unborn children have been recognized as acquiring rights or interests by way of inheritance or other devolution of property, and have been represented by [legal representatives]. Perfection of the interests involved, again, has generally been contingent upon live birth. In short, the unborn have never been recognized in the law as persons in the whole sense.

In view of all this, we do not agree that, by adopting one theory of life, Texas may override the rights of the pregnant woman that are at stake. We repeat, however, that the State does have an important and legitimate interest in preserving and protecting the health of the pregnant woman, whether she be a resident of the State or a nonresident who seeks medical consultation and treatment there, and that it has still *another* important and legitimate interest in protecting the potentiality of human life. These interests are separate and distinct. Each grows in substantiality as the woman approaches term and, at a point during pregnancy, each becomes "compelling."

236

Appendix

With respect to the State's important and legitimate interest in the health of the mother, the "compelling" point, in the light of present medical knowledge, is at approximately the end of the first trimester. This is so because of the now-established medical fact that until the end of the first trimester mortality in abortion may be less than mortality in normal childbirth. It follows that, from and after this point, a State may regulate the abortion procedure to the extent that the regulation reasonably relates to the preservation and protection of maternal health. Examples of permissible state regulation in this area are requirements as to the qualifications of the person who is to perform the abortion; as to the licensure of the person; as to the facility in which the procedure is to be performed, that is, whether it must be a hospital or may be a clinic or some other place of less-than-hospital status; as to the licensing of the facility; and the like.

This means, on the other hand, that, for the period of pregnancy prior to this "compelling" point, the attending physician, in consultation with his patient, is free to determine, without regulation by the State, that, in his medical judgment, the patient's pregnancy should be terminated. If that decision is reached, the judgment may be effectuated by an abortion free of interference by the State.

With respect to the State's important and legitimate interest in potential life, the "compelling" point is at viability. This is so because the fetus then presumably has the capability of meaningful life outside the mother's womb. State regulation protective of fetal life after viability thus has both logical and biological justifications. If the State is interested in protecting fetal life after viability, it may go so far as to proscribe [prohibit] abortion during that period, except when it is necessary to preserve the life or health of the mother.

Measured against these standards, [Article] 1196 of the Texas Penal Code, in restricting legal abortions to those "procured or attempted by medical advice for the purpose of saving the life of the mother," sweeps too broadly. The statute makes no distinction between abortions performed early in pregnancy and those performed later, and it limits to a single reason, "saving" the mother's life, the legal justification for the procedure. The statute, therefore, cannot survive the constitutional attack made upon it here . . .

To summarize and to repeat:

1. A state criminal abortion statute of the current Texas type, that excepts from criminality only a *lifesaving* procedure on behalf of the mother, without regard to pregnancy stage and without recognition of the other interests involved, is violative of the Due Process Clause of the Fourteenth Amendment.

(a) For the stage prior to approximately the end of the first trimester, the abortion decision and its effectuation must be left to the medical judgment of the pregnant woman's attending physician.

(b) For the stage subsequent to approximately the end of the first trimester, the State, in promoting its interest in the health of the mother, may, if it chooses, regulate the abortion procedure in ways that are reasonably related to maternal health.

(c) For the stage subsequent to viability, the State in promoting its interest in the potentiality of human life may, if it chooses, regulate, and even proscribe, abortion except where it is necessary, in appropriate medical judgment, for the preservation of the life or health of the mother.

2. The State may define the term "physician" . . . to mean only a physician currently licensed by the State, and may proscribe any abortion by a person who is not a physician as so defined . . .

This holding, we feel, is consistent with the relative weights of the respective interests involved, with the lessons and examples of medical and legal history, with the lenity of the common law, and with the demands of the profound problems of the present day. The decision leaves the State free to place increasing restrictions on abortion as the period of pregnancy lengthens, so long as those restrictions are tailored to the recognized state interests. The decision vindicates the right of the physician to administer medical treatment according to his professional judgment up to the points where important state interests provide compelling justifications for intervention. Up to those points, the abortion decision in all its aspects is inherently, and primarily, a medical decision, and basic responsibility for it must rest with the physician. If an individual practitioner abuses the privilege of exercising proper medical judgment, the usual remedies, judicial and intra-professional, are available.

Our conclusion that [Article] 1196 is unconstitutional means, of course, that the Texas abortion statutes, as a unit, must fall . . .

CHIEF JUSTICE BURGER, concurring: I agree that, under the Fourteenth Amendment to the Constitution, the abortion statues of Georgia and Texas impermissibly limit the performance of abortions necessary to protect the health of pregnant women, using the term health in its broadest medical context. I am somewhat troubled that the Court has taken notice of various scientific and medical data in reaching its conclusion; however, I do not believe that the Court has exceeded the scope of judicial notice accepted in other contexts.

In oral argument, counsel for the State of Texas informed the Court that Early abortive procedures were routinely permitted in certain exceptional cases, such as nonconsensual pregnancies resulting from rape and incest. In the face of a rigid and narrow statute, such as that of Texas, no one in these circumstances should be placed in a posture of dependence on a prosecutorial policy or prosecutorial discretion. Of course, States must have broad power, within the limits indicated in the opinions, to regulate the subject of abortions, but where the consequences of state intervention are so severe, uncertainty must be avoided as much as possible. For my part, I would be inclined to allow a State to require the certification of two physicians to support an abortion, but the Court holds otherwise. I do not believe that such a procedure is unduly burdensome, as are the complex steps of the Georgia statute [in *Doe v. Bolton*], which require as many as six doctors and the use of a hospital certified by the JCAH.

I do not read the Court's holdings today as having the sweeping consequences attributed to them by the dissenting Justices; the dissenting views discount the reality that the vast majority of physicians observe the standards of their profession, and act only on the basis of carefully deliberated medical judgements relating to life and health. Plainly, the Court today rejects any claim that the Constitution requires abortion on demand.

JUSTICE DOUGLAS, concurring [This opinion also applies to *Doe v. Bolton*]: While I join the opinion of the Court, I add a few words.

The questions presented in the present cases go far beyond the issues of vagueness, which we considered in *United States v. Vuitch*. They involve the right of privacy, one aspect of which we considered in *Griswold v. Connecticut*, when we held that various guarantees in the Bill of Rights create zones of privacy.

The *Griswold* case involved a law forbidding the use of contraceptives. We held that law as applied to married people unconstitutional:

"We deal with a right of privacy older than the Bill of Rights—older than our political parties, older than our school system. Marriage is a coming together for better or for worse, hopefully enduring, and intimate to the degree of being sacred."

The District Court in *Doe* held that *Griswold* and related cases "establish a Constitutional right to privacy broad enough to encompass the right of a woman to terminate an unwanted pregnancy in its early stages, by obtaining an abortion."

The Supreme Court of California expressed the same view in *People v. Belous*.

The Ninth Amendment obviously does not create federally enforceable rights. It merely says, "The enumeration in the Constitution, of certain rights, shall not be construed to deny or disparage others retained by the people." But a catalogue of these rights includes customary, traditional, and time-honored rights, amenities, privileges, and immunities that come within the sweep of "the Blessings of Liberty" mentioned in the preamble to the Constitution. Many of them, in my view, come within the meaning of the term "liberty" as used in the Fourteenth Amendment.

Reproductive Rights and Technology

First is the autonomous control over the development and expression of one's intellect, interests, tastes, and personality.

These are rights protected by the First Amendment and, in my view, they are absolute, permitting of no exceptions. The Free Exercise Clause of the First Amendment is one facet of this constitutional right. The right to remain silent as respects one's own beliefs is protected by the First and the Fifth. The First Amendment grants the privacy of first-class mail. All of these aspects of the right of privacy are rights "retained by the people" in the meaning of the Ninth Amendment.

Second is freedom of choice in the basic decisions of one's life respecting marriage, divorce, procreation, contraception, and the education and upbringing of children.

These rights, unlike those protected by the First Amendment, are subject to some control by the police power. Thus, the Fourth Amendment speaks only of "unreasonable searches and seizures" and of "probable cause." These rights are "fundamental," and we have held that in order to support legislative action the statute must be narrowly and precisely drawn and that a "compelling state interest" must be shown in support of the limitation.

The liberty to marry a person of one's own choosing; the right of procreation; the liberty to direct the education of one's children; and the privacy of the marital relation are in this category. Only last Term in *Eisenstadt v. Baird*, another contraceptive case, we expanded the concept of *Griswold* by saying:

"It is true that in *Griswold* the right of privacy in question inhered in the marital relationship. Yet the marital couple is not an independent entity with a mind and heart of its own, but an association of two individuals each with a separate intellectual and emotional makeup. If the right of privacy means anything, it is the right of the *individual*, married or single, to be free from unwarranted governmental intrusion into matters so fundamentally affecting a person as the decision whether to bear or beget a child."

This right of privacy was called by Justice Brandeis the right "to be let alone." That right includes the privilege of an individual to plan his own affairs, for, "'outside areas of plainly harmful conduct, every American is left to shape his own life as he thinks best, do what he pleases, go where he pleases.'"

Third is the freedom to care for one's health and person, freedom from bodily restraint or compulsion, freedom to walk, stroll, or loaf.

These rights, though fundamental, are likewise subject to regulation on a showing of "compelling state interest." We stated in *Papachristou v. City of Jacksonville* that walking, strolling, and wandering "are historically part of the amenities of life as we have know them." As stated in *Jacobson v. Massachusetts.*

"There is, of course, a sphere within which the individual may assert the supremacy of his own will and rightfully dispute the authority of any human

240

government, especially of any free government existing under a written constitution, to interfere with the exercise of that will."

. . . In *Terry v. Ohio*, the Court, in speaking of the Fourth Amendment,
stated, "This inestimable right of personal security belongs as much to the
citizen on the streets of our cities as to the homeowner closeted in his study
to dispose of his secret affairs."
. . . In *Meyer v. Nebraska*, the Court said:

*"Without doubt, it [liberty] denotes not merely freedom from bodily restraint
but also the right of the individual to contract, to engage in any of the common occupations of life, to acquire useful knowledge, to marry, establish a
home and bring up children, to worship God according to the dictates of his
own conscience, and generally to enjoy those privileges long recognized at common law as essential to the orderly pursuit of happiness by free men."*

The Georgia statute is at war with the clear message of these cases—that
a woman is free to make the basic decision whether to bear an unwanted
child. Elaborate argument is hardly necessary to demonstrate that childbirth
may deprive a woman of her preferred lifestyle and force upon her a radically different and undesired future. For example, rejected applicants under
the Georgia statute are required to endure the discomforts of pregnancy; to
incur the pain, higher mortality rate, and aftereffects of childbirth; to aban-
don educational plans; to sustain loss of income; to forgo the satisfactions of
careers; to tax further mental and physical health in providing child care;
and, in some cases, to bear the lifelong stigma of unwed motherhood, a
badge which may haunt, if not deter, later legitimate family relationships.
     Such reasoning is, however, only the beginning of the problem. The
State has interests to protect. Vaccinations to prevent epidemics are one example, as *Jacobson* holds. The Court held that compulsory sterilization of
imbeciles afflicted with hereditary forms of insanity or imbecility is another.
Abortion affects another. While childbirth endangers the lives of some
women, voluntary abortion at any time and place regardless of medical standards would impinge on a rightful concern of society. The woman's health
is part of that concern; as is the life of the fetus after quickening. These concerns justify the State in treating the procedure as a medical one.
     One difficulty is that this statute as construed and applied apparently
does not give full sweep to the "psychological as well as physical well-being"
of women patients which saved the concept "health" from being void for
vagueness in *United States v. Vuitch*. But, apart from that, Georgia's enactment has a constitutional infirmity because . . . it "limits the number of reasons for which an abortion may be sought." I agree with the holding of the

District Court, "This the State may not do, because such action unduly restricts a decision sheltered by the Constitutional right to privacy."

The vicissitudes of life produce pregnancies which may be unwanted, or which may impair "health" in the broad *Vuitch* sense of the term, or which may imperil the life of the mother, or which in the full setting of the case may create such suffering, dislocations, misery, or tragedy as to make an early abortion the only civilized step to take. These hardships may be properly embraced in the "health" factor of the mother as appraised by a person of insight. Or they may be part of a broader medical judgment based on what is "appropriate" in a given case, though perhaps not "necessary" in a strict sense.

The "liberty" of the mother, though rooted as it is in the Constitution, may be qualified by the State for the reasons we have stated. But where fundamental personal rights and liberties are involved, the corrective legislation must be "narrowly drawn to prevent the supposed evil," and not be dealt with in an "unlimited and indiscriminate" manner. Unless regulatory measures are so confined and are addressed to the specific areas of compelling legislative concern, the police power would become the great leveler of constitutional rights and liberties.

There is no doubt that the State may require abortions to be performed by qualified medical personnel. The legitimate objective of preserving the mother's health clearly supports such laws. Their impact upon the woman's privacy is minimal. But the Georgia statute outlaws virtually all such operations—even in the earliest stages of pregnancy. In light of modern medical evidence suggesting that an early abortion is safer healthwise than childbirth itself, it cannot be seriously urged that so comprehensive a ban is aimed at protecting the woman's health. Rather, this expansive proscription of all abortions along the temporal spectrum can rest only on a public goal of preserving both embryonic and fetal life.

The present statute has struck the balance between the woman's and the State's interests wholly in favor of the latter. I am not prepared to hold that a State may equate, as Georgia has done, all phases of maturation preceding birth. We held in *Griswold* that the States may not preclude spouses from attempting to avoid the joinder of sperm and egg. If this is true, it is difficult to perceive any overriding public necessity which might attach precisely at the moment of conception. As Justice Clark has said:

> *"To say that life is present at conception is to give recognition to the potential, rather than the actual. The unfertilized egg has life, and if fertilized, it takes on human proportions. But the law deals in reality, not obscurity—the known rather than the unknown. When sperm meets egg life may eventually form, but quite often it does not. The law does not deal in speculation. The phe-*

Appendix

nomenon of life takes time to develop, and until it is actually present, it cannot be destroyed. Its interruption prior to formation would hardly be homicide, and as we have seen, society does not regard it as such. The rites of Baptism are not performed and death certificates are not required when a miscarriage occurs. No prosecutor has ever returned a murder indictment charging the taking of the life of a fetus. This would not be the case if the fetus constituted human life."

In summary, the enactment is overbroad. It is not closely correlated to the aim of preserving prenatal life. In fact, it permits its destruction in several cases, including pregnancies resulting from sex acts in which unmarried females are below the statutory age of consent. At the same time, however, the measure broadly proscribes aborting other pregnancies which may cause severe mental disorders. Additionally, the statute is overbroad because it equates the value of embryonic life immediately after conception with the worth of life immediately before birth.

Under the Georgia Act, the mother's physician is not the sole judge as to whether the abortion should be performed. Two other licensed physicians must concur in his judgment. Moreover, the abortion must be performed in a licensed hospital; and the abortion must be approved in advance by a committee of the medical staff of the hospital.

Physicians . . . complain of the Georgia Act's interference with their practice of their profession.

The right of privacy has no more conspicuous place than in the physician-patient relationship, unless it be in the priest-penitent relation.

It is one thing for a patient to agree that her physician may consult with another physician about her case. It is quite a different matter for the State compulsorily to impose on that physician-patient relationship another layer or, as in this case, still a third layer of physicians. The right of privacy—the right to care for one's health and person and to seek out a physician of one's own choice protected by the Fourteenth Amendment—becomes only a matter of theory, not a reality, when a multiple-physician-approval system is mandated by the State.

The State licenses a physician. If he is derelict or faithless, the procedures available to punish him or to deprive him of his license are well known. He is entitled to procedural due process before professional disciplinary sanctions may be imposed. Crucial here, however, is state-imposed control over the medical decision whether pregnancy should be interrupted. The good-faith decision of the patient's chosen physician is overridden and the final decision passed on to others in whose selection the patient has no part. This is a total destruction of the right of privacy between physician and patient and the intimacy of relation which that entails.

The right to seek advice on one's health and the right to place reliance on the physician of one's choice are basic to Fourteenth Amendment values. We deal with fundamental rights and liberties, which, as already noted, can be contained or controlled only by discretely drawn legislation that preserves the "liberty" and regulates only those phases of the problem of compelling legislative concern. The imposition by the State of group controls over the physician-patient relationship is not made on any medical procedure apart from abortion, no matter how dangerous the medical step may be. The oversight imposed on the physician and patient in abortion cases denies them their "liberty," [that is,] their right of privacy, without any compelling, discernible state interest.

Georgia has constitutional warrant in treating abortion as a medical problem. To protect the woman's right of privacy, however, the control must be through the physician of her choice and the standards set for his performance.

The protection of the fetus when it has acquired life is a legitimate concern of the State. Georgia's law makes no rational, discernible decision on that score. For under the Code, the developmental stage of the fetus is irrelevant when pregnancy is the result of rape, when the fetus will very likely be born with a permanent defect, or when a continuation of the pregnancy will endanger the life of the mother or permanently injure her health. When life is present is a question we do not try to resolve. While basically a question for medical experts, . . . it is, of course, caught up in matters of religion and morality.

In short, I agree with the Court that endangering the life of the woman or seriously and permanently injuring her health are standards too narrow for the right of privacy that is at stake.

I also agree that the superstructure of medical supervision which Georgia has erected violates the patient's right of privacy inherent in her choice of her own physician.

JUSTICE STEWART, concurring: In 1963, this Court, in *Ferguson v. Skrupa*, purported to sound the death knell for the doctrine of substantive due process, a doctrine under which many state laws had in the past been held to violate the Fourteenth Amendment. As Justice Black's opinion for the Court in *Skrupa* put it: "We have returned to the original constitutional proposition that courts do not substitute their social and economic beliefs for the judgment of legislative bodies, who are elected to pass laws."

Barely two years later, in *Griswold v. Connecticut*, the Court held a Connecticut birth control law unconstitutional. . . . [I]t was clear to me then, and it is equally clear to me now, that the *Griswold* decision can be rationally understood only as a holding that the Connecticut statute substantively invaded the "liberty" that is protected by the Due Process Clause of the

Appendix

Fourteenth Amendment. As so understood, *Griswold* stands as one in a long line of pre-*Skrupa* cases decided under the doctrine of substantive due process, and I now accept it as such.

"In a Constitution for a free people, there can be no doubt that the meaning of 'liberty' must be broad indeed." The Constitution nowhere mentions a specific right of personal choice in matters of marriage and family life, but the "liberty" protected by the Due Process Clause of the Fourteenth Amendment covers more than those freedoms explicitly named in the Bill of Rights.

As Justice Harlan once wrote: "[T]he full scope of the liberty guaranteed by the Due Process Clause cannot be found in or limited by the precise terms of the specific guarantees elsewhere provided in the Constitution. This 'liberty' is not a series of isolated points pricked out in terms of the taking of property; the freedom of speech, press, and religion; the right to keep and bear arms; the freedom from unreasonable searches and seizures; and so on. It is a rational continuum which, broadly speaking, includes a freedom from all substantial arbitrary impositions and purposeless restraints . . . and which also recognizes, what a reasonable and sensitive judgment must, that certain interests require particularly careful scrutiny of the state needs asserted to justify their abridgment." In the words of Justice Frankfurter, "Great concepts like . . . 'liberty' . . . were purposely left to gather meaning from experience. For they relate to the whole domain of social and economic fact, and the statesmen who founded this Nation knew too well that only a stagnant society remains unchanged."

Several decisions of this Court make clear that freedom of personal choice in matters of marriage and family life is one of the liberties protected by the Due Process Clause of the Fourteenth Amendment. As recently as last Term, in *Eisenstadt v. Baird*, we recognized "the right of the *individual*, married or single, to be free from unwarranted governmental intrusion into matters so fundamentally affecting a person as the decision whether to bear or beget a child." That right necessarily includes the right of a woman to decide whether or not to terminate her pregnancy. "Certainly the interests of a woman in giving of her physical and emotional self during pregnancy and the interests that will be affected throughout her life by the birth and raising of a child are of a far greater degree of significance and personal intimacy than the right to send a child to private school protected in *Pierce v. Society of Sisters*, or the right to teach a foreign language protected in *Meyer v. Nebraska*.

Clearly, therefore, the Court today is correct in holding that the right asserted by Jane Roe is embraced within the personal liberty protected by the Due Process Clause of the Fourteenth Amendment.

It is evident that the Texas abortion statute infringes that right directly. Indeed, it is difficult to imagine a more complete abridgment of a constitutional freedom than that worked by the inflexible criminal statute now in force in Texas. The question then becomes whether the state interests advanced to justify this abridgment can survive the "particularly careful scrutiny" that the Fourteenth Amendment here requires.

The asserted state interests are protection of the health and safety of the pregnant woman, and protection of the potential future human life within her. These are legitimate objectives, amply sufficient to permit a State to regulate abortions as it does other surgical procedures, and perhaps sufficient to permit a State to regulate abortions more stringently or even to prohibit them in the late stages of pregnancy. But such legislation is not before us, and I think the Court today has thoroughly demonstrated that these state interests cannot constitutionally support the broad abridgment of personal liberty worked by the existing Texas law. Accordingly, I join the Court's opinion holding that that law is invalid under the Due Process Clause of the Fourteenth Amendment.

JUSTICE WHITE (joined by Justice Rehnquist), dissenting [This opinion also applies to *Doe v. Bolton*]: At the heart of the controversy in these cases are those recurring pregnancies that pose no danger whatsoever to the life or health of the mother but are, nevertheless, unwanted for any one or more of a variety of reasons—convenience, family planning, economics, dislike of children, the embarrassment of illegitimacy, etc. The common claim before us is that for any one of such reasons, or for no reason at all, and without asserting or claiming any threat to life or health, any woman is entitled to an abortion at her request if she is able to find a medical advisor willing to undertake the procedure.

The Court for the most part sustains this position: During the period prior to the time the fetus becomes viable, the Constitution of the United States values the convenience, whim, or caprice of the putative mother more than the life or potential life of the fetus; the Constitution, therefore, guarantees the right to an abortion as against any state law or policy seeking to protect the fetus from an abortion not prompted by more compelling reasons of the mother.

With all due respect, I dissent. I find nothing in the language or history of the Constitution to support the Court's judgment. The Court simply fashions and announces a new constitutional right for pregnant mothers and, with scarcely any reason or authority for its action, invests that right with sufficient substance to override most existing state abortion statutes. The upshot is that the people and the legislatures of the 50 States are constitutionally disentitled to weigh the relative importance of the continued existence and development of the fetus, on the one hand, against a spectrum of possible impacts on the mother, on the other hand. As an exercise of raw judicial power, the Court perhaps has authority to do what it does today; but in my view its judgment is an improvident and extravagant exercise of the power of judicial review that the Constitution extends to this Court.

The Court apparently values the convenience of the pregnant mother more than the continued existence and development of the life or potential life that she carries. Whether or not I might agree with that marshaling of values, I can in no event join the Court's judgment because I find no constitutional warrant for imposing such an order of priorities on the people and legislatures of the States. In a sensitive area such as this, involving as it does issues over which reasonable men may easily and heatedly differ, I cannot accept the Court's exercise of its clear power of choice by interposing a constitutional barrier to state efforts to protect human life and by investing mothers and doctors with the constitutionally protected right to exterminate it. This issue, for the most part, should be left with the people and to the political processes the people have devised to govern their affairs.

It is my view, therefore, that the Texas statute is not constitutionally infirm because it denies abortions to those who seek to serve only their convenience rather than to protect their life or health. Nor is this plaintiff, who claims no threat to her mental or physical health, entitled to assert the possible rights of those women whose pregnancy assertedly implicates their health . . .

I would reverse the judgment of the District Court in the Georgia case.

JUSTICE WILLIAM REHNQUIST, dissenting: The Court's opinion brings to the decision of this troubling question both extensive historical fact and a wealth of legal scholarship. While the opinion thus commands my respect, I find myself nonetheless in fundamental disagreement with those parts of it that invalidate the Texas statute in question, and therefore dissent.

The Court's opinion decides that a State may impose virtually no restriction on the performance of abortions during the first trimester of pregnancy. Our previous decisions indicate that a necessary predicate for such an opinion is a plaintiff who was in her first trimester of pregnancy at some time during the pendency of her lawsuit. While a party may vindicate his own constitutional rights, he may not seek vindication for the rights of others. The Court's statement of facts in this case makes clear, however, that the record in no way indicates the presence of such a plaintiff. We know only the plaintiff Roe at the time of filing her complaint was a pregnant woman; for aught that appears in this record, she may have been in her *last* trimester of pregnancy as of the date the complaint was filed.

Nothing in the Court's opinion indicates that Texas might not constitutionally apply its proscription of abortion as written to a woman in that stage of pregnancy. Nonetheless, the Court uses her complaint against the Texas statute as a fulcrum for deciding that States may impose virtually no restrictions on medical abortions performed during the *first* trimester of pregnancy. In deciding such a hypothetical lawsuit, the Court departs from the long-standing admonition that it should never "formulate a rule of constitutional law broader than is required by the precise facts to which it is to be applied."

Even if there were a plaintiff in this case capable of litigating the issue which the Court decides, I would reach a conclusion opposite to that reached by the Court. I have difficulty in concluding, as the Court does, that the right of "privacy" is involved in this case. Texas, by the statute here challenged, bars the performance of a medical abortion by a licensed physician on a plaintiff such as Roe. A transaction resulting in an operation such as this is not "private" in the ordinary usage of that word. Nor is the "privacy" that the Court finds here even a distant relative of the freedom from searches and seizures protected by the Fourth Amendment to the Constitution, which the Court has referred to as embodying a right to privacy.

If the Court means by the term "privacy" no more than that the claim of a person to be free from unwanted state regulation of consensual transactions may be a form of "liberty" protected by the Fourteenth Amendment, there is no doubt that similar claims have been upheld in our earlier decisions on the basis of that liberty. I agree with the statement of Justice Stewart in his concurring opinion that the "liberty," against deprivation of which without due process the Fourteenth Amendment protects, embraces more than the rights found in the Bill of Rights. But that liberty is not guaranteed absolutely against deprivation, only against deprivation without due process of law. The test traditionally applied in the area of social and economic legislation is whether or not a law such as that challenged has a rational relation to a valid state objective. The Due Process Clause of the Fourteenth Amendment undoubtedly does place a limit, albeit a broad one, on legislative power to enact laws such as this. If the Texas statute were to prohibit an abortion even where the mother's life is in jeopardy, I have little doubt that such a statute would lack a rational relation to a valid state objective under the test stated in *Williamson*. But the Court's sweeping invalidation of any restrictions on abortion during the first trimester is impossible to justify under that standard, and the conscious weighing of competing factors that the Court's opinion apparently substitutes for the established test is far more appropriate to a legislative judgment than to a judicial one.

The Court eschews the history of the Fourteenth Amendment in its reliance on the "compelling state interest" test. But the Court adds a new wrinkle to this test by transposing it from the legal considerations associated with the Equal Protection Clause of the Fourteenth Amendment to this case arising under the Due Process Clause of the Fourteenth Amendment. Unless I misapprehend the consequences of this transplanting of the "compelling state interest test," the Court's opinion will accomplish the seemingly impossible feat of leaving this area of the law more confused than it found it.

. . . As in *Lochner [v. New York]* and similar cases applying substantive due process standards to economic and social welfare legislation, the adoption of the compelling state interest standard will inevitably require this Court to examine the legislative policies and pass on the wisdom of these policies in the very process of deciding whether a particular state interest put forward may or may not be "compelling." The decision here to break pregnancy into three distinct terms and to outline the permissible restrictions the State may impose in each one, for example, partakes more of judicial legislation than it does of a determination of the intent of the drafters of the Fourteenth Amendment.

The fact that a majority of the States reflecting, after all, the majority sentiment in those States, have had restrictions on abortions for at least a century is a strong indication, it seems to me, that the asserted right to an abortion is not "so rooted in the traditions and conscience of our people as to be ranked as fundamental." Even today, when society's views on abortion are changing, the very existence of the debate is evidence that the "right" to an abortion is not so universally accepted as [Roe] would have us believe.

To reach its result the Court necessarily has had to find within the scope of the Fourteenth Amendment a right that was apparently completely unknown to the drafters of the Amendment. As early as 1821, the first state law dealing directly with abortion was enacted by the Connecticut Legislature. By the time of the adoption of the Fourteenth Amendment in 1868, there were at least 36 laws enacted by state or territorial legislatures limiting abortion. While many States have amended or updated their laws, 21 of the laws on the books in 1868 remain in effect today. Indeed, the Texas statute struck down today was, as the majority notes, first enacted in 1857 and "has remained substantially unchanged to the present time."

There apparently was no question concerning the validity of this provision or of any of the other state statutes when the Fourteenth Amendment was adopted. The only conclusion possible from this history is that the drafters did not intend to have the Fourteenth Amendment withdraw from the States the power to legislate with respect to this matter.

Even if one were to agree that the case that the Court decides were here, and that the enunciation of the substantive constitutional law in the Court's opinion were proper, the actual disposition of the case by the Court is still difficult to justify. The Texas statute is struck down in toto, even though the Court apparently concedes that at later periods of pregnancy Texas might impose these selfsame statutory limitations on abortion. My understanding of past practice is that a statute found to be invalid as applied to a particular plaintiff, but no unconstitutional as a whole, is not simply "struck down" but is, instead, declared unconstitutional as applied to the fact situation before the Court.

For all of the foregoing reasons, I respectfully dissent.

INDEX

Index locators in **boldface** indicate main topics.

251

Index

Index

Index